This book is dedicated to those who have gone before us and on whose shoulders, we now stand; we now hold the baton and are determined to carry it to the finish line. It is also lasting tribute to the NHS of which we are incredibly grateful and proud.

Caribbeans Recruited to Serve
Copyright © 2020

All rights reserved. No part of this publication may be reproduced, stored in a retrieval system or transmitted in any form or by any means, electronic, mechanical, photocopying, recording or otherwise, without written permission from Barbados Overseas Nurses Association UK or in accordance with the permission of the Copyright Act 1956. Any person or persons who do any unauthorised act in relation to this publication may be liable to criminal prosecution and civil claims for damages.

Contents Page

Foreword
Author/Compiler's note
First President, Pauline Sealy
S. Peters
B. Brewster MBE JP
O. Weekes
N. Redwood-Sawyerr
G. Redwood-Sawyerr
Julia Alleyne
H. Marshall
C. Goodman
M. Morris-Springer
Maria Layne-Springer
Angela Alleyne
Reflective Photos
S. Clarke
Waple's Story
Dalton McConney MBE QPM Patron
C. De Abreau
Presentation
Lorraine Whitehall
Marie Greenidge
Monica Gordon
Harold Springer
Gloria Gittens
Carmita Neblett
Golda Griffith, Cecelia Rodrigues
Rev. Jackie's Journey
Jean Miller, Joan Bynoe-Saul, Phyllis Chase
Recipients of our Fundraising effort
Tributes: Herbert (Herbie) E. Yearwood DHC 1995-2008 Anthony Sandiford WIIFA, Esther Holmes MBE Rev David A. Hoyte, Rev Rosemary Taylor.

Foreword

I am delighted to write the foreword to this journal on the experiences of individuals, mainly nurses, who were recruited from Barbados during the early sixties and the seventies. These individuals, now known as the Windrush Generation, contributed significantly to the social and economic development of the United Kingdom.

The void created because of the Second World War, demanded the recruitment of Caribbean workers to supplement the depleted workforce. Many people, most of whom were nurses, arrived in the United Kingdom to help with the establishment of the National Health Service.

As we read this journal and reminisce on the struggles and achievements of the past, we can certainly say with pride that we have fought and won the good fight. We also unanimously agree that the great contributions we have made through our hard work, dedication and commitment to the job, could not have been possible without the unstinting financial, emotional and physical support of our partners who were the backbone of our efforts. In retrospect, we know that we could not have persevered without them and wonder whether the NHS would have survived without our contributions.

Barbara Brewster MBE JP President 1997 – 2000

Compiler's Comments

As Secretary of Barbados Overseas Nurses Association (B.O.N.A), I agreed to compile these stories into this book which intend to closely examine and construct a historical record of the relationships and experiences of these young men and women, some just out of school who embarked on a journey to a far-away country and train as nurses, not knowing what was awaiting them at the other destination. The title of the book is in relation to our motto "To Serve" and being part of the solution. Members had already been made aware of the importance of recording their journeys in the NHS and as Secretary I was present at the initial consultations. I am especially honoured to be compiling the various accounts of their remarkable and individual stories which highlighted the pitfalls, the challenges, their experiences and achievements in the medical profession, despite at times encountering inappropriate hostility. The purpose of this book is to enlighten the reader about the significant contribution of the nurses to the growth and major success of the NHS which reached its 70th year (2018); this of course stimulated feelings of urgency in the members who then set a target date for the completion of the book in the 25th. year of their anniversary. Finally, we are grateful for the insight of the six nurses, namely: Pauline Sealy, Iona Gittens, Sheila Atherley, Jennifer Howell, Carlma DeAbreau and Oriel Weekes who initiated the birth of B.O.N.A in February 1994. This organisation enabled them, with the support of their husbands, partners, family, and friends to use their expertise in establishing a social and welfare mechanism, in support of their fundraising efforts for various charities in Barbados and the UK.

Ceifred Goodman

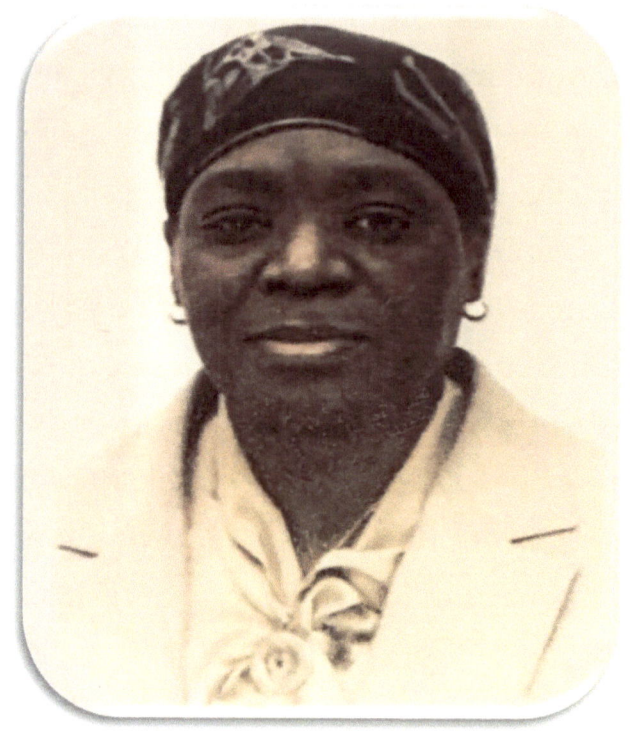

Mrs. Pauline Sealy, 1st. President

"I'd like the memory of me to be a happy one
I'd like to leave an afterglow of smiles when
my life is done.

My Journey Through The NHS

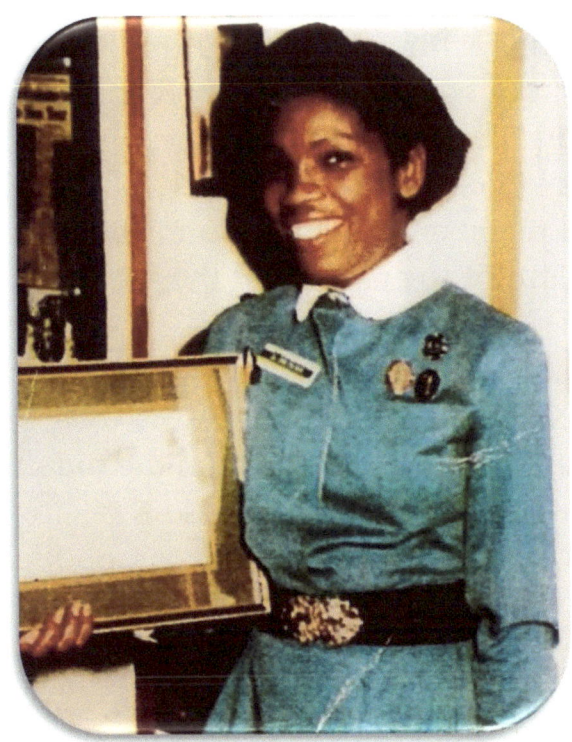

Shermane Peters

I am one of a group of Barbadians who were recruited directly from school to train as Nurses in the United Kingdom, "Mother Country", back in the late sixties. This was the result of a delegation of health Professionals who came from the UK to the Caribbean with a clear mission to recruit as many young adults to take up a career in Nursing and then to work at the various hospitals across the UK.

In the case of many Barbadians, the process involved the Barbados Government. Through the Employment Exchange, we had to undergo stringent health checks, including immunisation to certify that we were fit to travel and take on the training. The Barbadian Government also paid for the flight tickets and the travel documents, but a family member took the responsibility and signed as guarantor to ensure that the money is repaid.

The plane flights at that time were full, approximately 250 young people were on the flight to take up various positions in the nursing profession; some to study and others to work at places like London Transport as Conductors and drivers, some to work in other establishments such as Lyons, Fords and Leyland's.

We, the student Nurses were paired up in sets 2 – 6 to go to various NHS hospitals across the UK. I went to the Southampton group of hospitals in Hampshire. I was paired up with another student. On arrival at Heathrow Airport, we were met by the British council staff who made us feel welcomed and they gave us directions on how to get to Southampton via Waterloo station. My sister who was unable to meet me sent her husband to ensure that I was warmly clad as it was December and to checked if I needed anything further.

On arrival in Southampton, we were taken by taxi to the Nurses home and there we were welcomed by the home warden, who ensured that we were made comfortable. We had a good orientation program around the nurse's home and the hospital wards. The home warden had delegated the hospital tour to be done by the Senior Students.

My career in Nursing commenced with the General training which took about four years, during which time I got married and had a son. I took maternity leave and resumed my nurse training after one year. I was determined to achieve my goal; I took my training seriously and gained my SRN certificate and badge. Although I trained as a nurse, my interest was always in Midwifery, so after a short break I applied for and gained a place to train as a midwife at Mayday Hospital in Croydon Surrey. The training then was in two parts part one and part two. Having successfully completed both, I applied for a midwife post and gained employment at Kings College Hospital (KCH) London.

At the end of the first year, I was promoted to a Midwifery sister and remained there from 1974-1985 because I got a lot of job satisfaction and the domestic location suited me. During those years I kept up to date by attending In-Service training and Mandatory Midwifery refresher Courses every five years. I also undertook the Family Planning course and did some sessions at the KCH Clinic. I also did the City and Guilds 730 Teaching Certificate.

I left KCH in 1985 for promotion to a Midwifery Manager's post in Charge of three postnatal wards at St. Heliers Hospital. During that time, I studied for the Certificate in Management Studies (CMS) and the Post-Graduate Diploma in Health Education (PGdp). This was truly relevant and an integral part of my role, because of the volume of nurses and medical students allocated to the ward and had to be taught and mentored.
Finally, I did my MSc in Health Education at Brunel University. Apart from keeping up to date, these further qualifications enabled me to take on other roles such as Supervisor of Midwives. This was a two-prong title, one aspect was to do with service provision, and the other side was checking that midwives kept up to date and were fit to practice.

My final appointment in the NHS was as a senior Community Midwife at Chelsea and Westminster hospital. I thoroughly enjoyed my work as a midwife and found it hard to leave.

Overall, I have had an incredibly positive experience since I came to England. I am not saying that there were no "bumpy rides" because I never personally experienced blatant racism. Yet the few times that I noticed it I found ways to manage it like diverting my energy in a more positive way.
I have three sons and I shared my experiences with them over the years. My late husband, Olu Peters, had always been incredibly supportive during my

career and post graduate studies; he also shared the domestic roles and took care of the boys.

With the birth of B.O.N.A 25 years ago, my sister Carlma De Abreau, one of the founder members of BONA, encouraged me to join the organisation. However, I did not join in the early years as I was too busy raising my family and doing my post graduate studies to enhance my role and keep up to date.

When I joined B.O.N.A, there were several posts to be taken. I agreed to be the Concert Co-Ordinator. B.O.N.A is a terribly busy organisation, participating in cultural trips, river cruises, variety concerts, banquets, sponsored walks, and recreation activities such as Line Dancing, exercises, quizzes, and game sessions annually. We also boast a 26-member choir where I was joined by my husband who played a significant role in the bass section. I keep fit by attending the gym. My hobbies include reading, painting, walking in the park and attending social events. I take holidays annually.

In conclusion I am now retired and have been elected as the President of B.O.N.A in June 2018, a position I am expected to occupy for the next two years. Now that the baton has been passed to me, I promised to perform my duties to the glory of God and the benefit of this association.

Barbara Brewster MBE JP

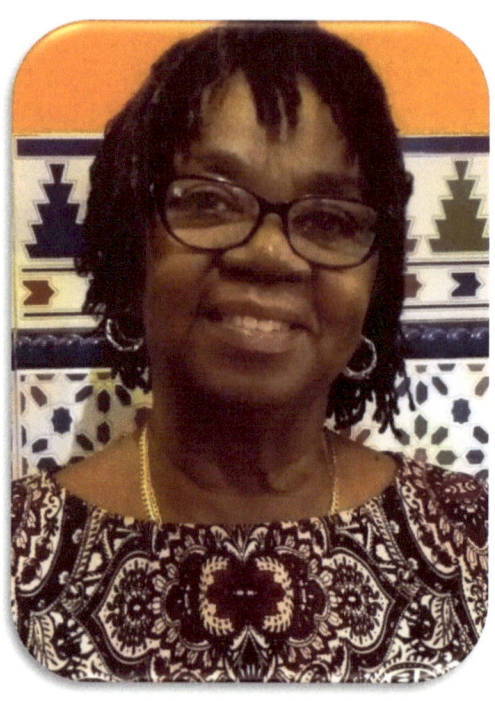

The invitation to contribute to the Barbados Overseas Nurses Association's journal celebrating its 25th anniversary, is indeed an honour which I eagerly and delightfully accepted. I was born in Barbados and travelled to England in the 1960's to train as a nurse and then a midwife.

I arrived in England on December 29th. 1964 four days after Christmas. I remember that day as vividly as though it was yesterday. It was a cold, dreary, winter's day; the antithesis of the sunny climes and warm inviting beaches of the homeland I had just left behind. However, my attention was caught by the beauty of the Christmas decorations along the streets and which hung from the tall buildings. These gave me a bit of comfort and a feeling of welcome in an otherwise seemingly dismal and depressing atmosphere. As I travelled along to my destination, outside became darker and darker.

I could not see the roads very clearly and a sense of dread filled me. I wondered to myself, what are you doing here in this strange place?

You did not have any family and only a few friends here in London. Do you really want to be here? I thought that I would wait until the next day and if anyone asked who wanted to return home to Barbados, I would be the first in line; wild horses would not stop me. I do not know how differently my life would have been because that question was never asked and forty-five years later, I was still in the UK; had achieved career success, married, raised a family and had quite settled into the English way of life.

Like all other immigrants, my journey to reach this point was filled with interesting challenges, highs and lows, ups and downs, but I am grateful that there have been more ups than downs.

When I first came to the UK, I wanted to join my friends to pursue training as a State Enrolled Nurse. However, I accepted some wise counsel that pointed me to a career path as a State Registered Nurse instead, which is a higher qualification. This was the best advice given and embraced as it stood me in good stead in the years to come. Thus, my journey to become an SRN and subsequently through the NHS began at the St. Nicholas Hospital and has been an exciting and challenging one. This journey has enabled me to achieve significantly while working in the NHS. I was able to complete a BSc. degree in Health Studies and an MSc in Health Promotion. Although I was trained as a midwife, midwifery was not my forte, therefore I practiced for only six months after qualifying and then returned to general nursing. This decision afforded me the opportunity over the years, to work in several London hospitals as a general nurse and led to my being appointed Night Sister at the then St. James Hospital in Balham, SW London, and later promoted to Night Services Manager at St George's Hospital, where I led a team of ten-night practitioners, before accepting early retirement in 1999. My training as a Registered Nurse and my degree qualifications certainly prepared me for and was instrumental in my gaining the post of Development Officer at the Sickle Cell Society. Although probably not connected, I believe my training as a Registered Nurse also positively influenced my appointment as a magistrate serving at the West London magistrate's court.

On reflection, at this point I am glad that the offer to return to Barbados was not asked in December 1964, because I surely would not have had the experiences which have shaped me into being the person I am today.

I take this opportunity to wish BONA heartiest congratulations on celebrating 25 years of service. I am indeed most grateful and privileged to have served as the Barbados Overseas Nurses Association's 2nd president for 2 terms: 1997 to 2000 and 2003 to 2006. As president I was privileged to lead BONA into the millennium, as we joined with the Barbados Registered Nurses Association in Barbados to celebrate Nurses' Week. My wish for BONA is that we go forward in love and grace remembering the words of Vince Lombardi, "The achievements of an organisation are the results of the combined effort of each individual."

Oriel Weekes, Founder Member

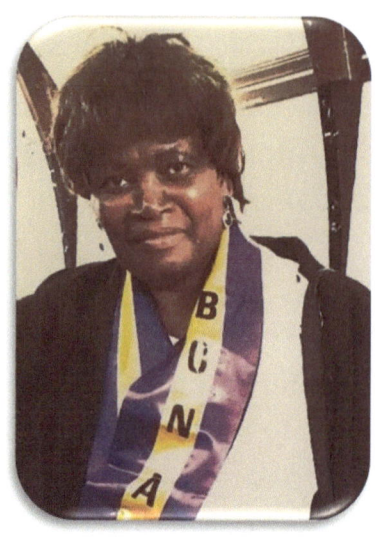

Fellow Barbadians and friends of B.O.N.A 25 years have flown by so quickly since the Association was formed in 1994. The Association was founded by Oriel Weekes, Iona Gittens, Pauline Sealey (who sadly died 2018) Jennifer Howell, Sheila Atherley and Carlma DeAbreau.

Our first meeting was held on the 4th. February 1994 at Parchmore Hall, Thornton Heath. Pauline chaired the meeting and Iona took the role of Secretary, Sheila became the Treasurer, Jennifer social Co-ordinator and Oriel the Public Relations Officer (PRO), Violet Legall was our first Vice President (who died in 1997). Our first launch and social party was held on Saturday the 3rd December 1994. BONA is a voluntary organisation and a charity whose objectives are to support its members, current and past, professionally; it also supports children's and other organisations both in the UK and Barbados through donations.

May I take this opportunity to thank God for BONA's Members, family friends and well-wishers for their continued support, time, and commitment. May the Organisation continue go on for many more years to come.

Norma Redwood-Sawyer

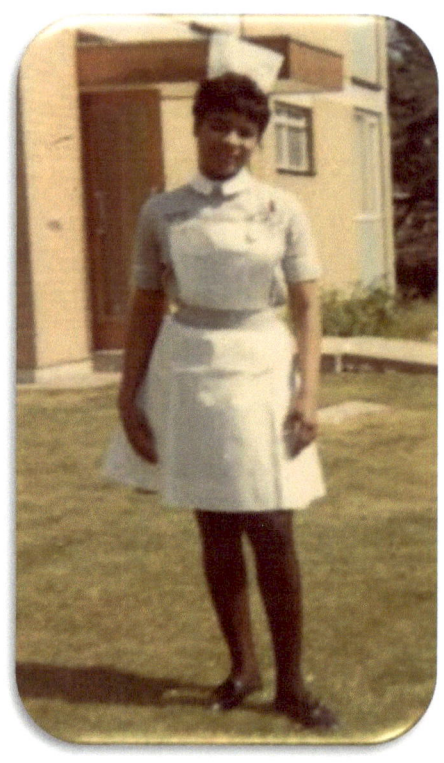

I arrived in England on the 24th June 1964, and started my training at Leicester Hillcrest hospital, completing at Mount Vernon Hospital, Middlesex. At the End of the training I gained my State Registered Nursing certificate. Did my part one Midwifery training at the Victoria Memorial Hospital and part two at Amersham Hospital. At the end of my training, I took a post as a midwife at Mayday Hospital in 1974 and remained there up until 2010 (36yrs). My first post was as a Staff Midwife, then Midwifery Sister and Acting Midwifery Manager. During those years, I did

Study days and Inservice training, Counseling and Communication Courses. I mentored student nurses, student Midwives and medical students. I had my daughter but continued my career with good support from my husband.

I joined B.O.N.A. in 1994 and was the social coordinator for several years. I enjoyed being a member of B.O.N.A and contributed to its growth up to 25 years. I am incredibly happy that it has reached this milestone.

Gladstone Redwood-Sawyerr

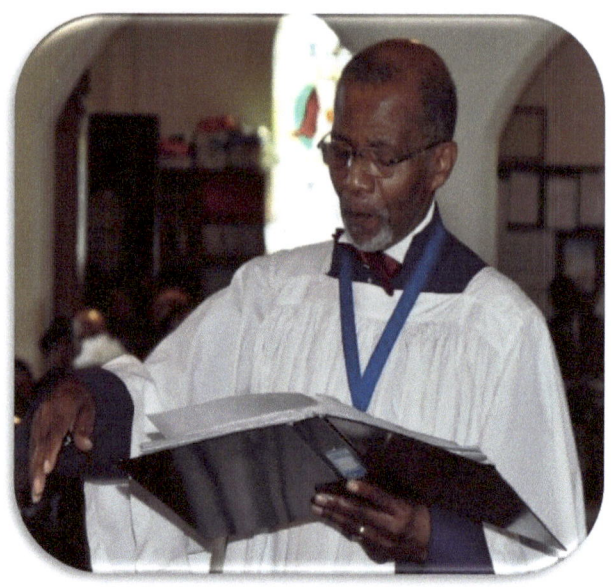

I came to England to further my career in nursing, having completed my training. I gained Employment at a hospital in Gloucestershire.

Later I did further studies and gained a BSc and MSc in nursing studies. These additional qualifications enabled me to take up a post at Kingston University, and senior lecture post at St Georges hospital.

I also mentored several students over the years.

I joined B.O.N.A initially to support my wife and the organisation later became a full member. I took an active role in the Church committee, and as a choir member, and Social committee. I also gave lectures on Mental health issues.

Julia Alleyne

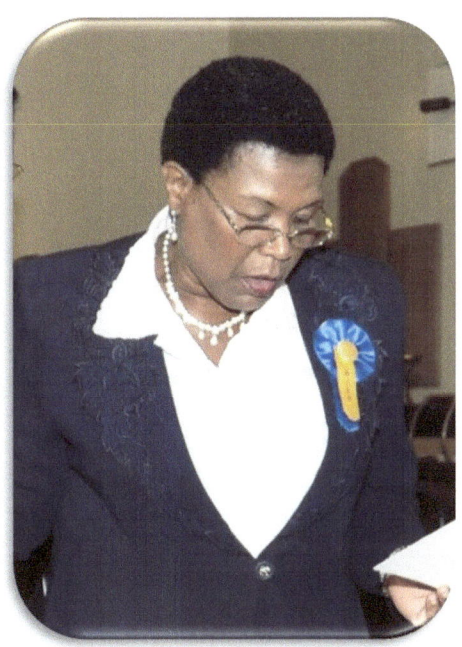

My Journey in the NHS

I came to England to pursue my Nursing career and at the end of the general nursing I did part one Midwifery training but did not do my part two, because I had a passion for Mental Health Nursing. I remained in that specialty for many years. I joined the London borough of Croydon as a Care Officer and then as an assistant residential Manager.

I joined B.O.N.A. soon after its Inception 1994, I took on various roles and finally was the treasurer for four terms (12) in which I enjoyed and gained good experience.

In 2012 I relocated to Barbados, but always remained a member of B.O.NA.

Hamilton Marshall

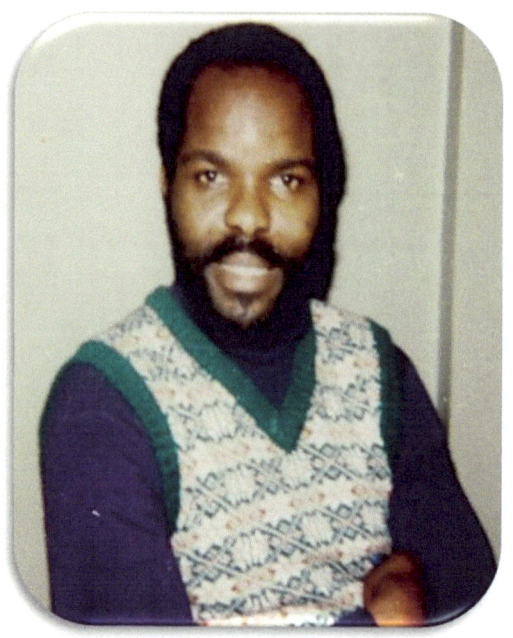

I attended West St Joseph Comprehensive School in Blackmans
St Joseph, (now Grantley Adams School). I was successful in passing my GCSE Certificates but first worked for Andrews Sugar Factory during the 1967 Crop season. My job was to weigh the sugar prior to it being transported to the Deep Water Harbour. At the end of the crop season, I went to the Ministry of Education – not knowing what I wanted to do. I met an Educator I knew from my School days and having told him that I was looking for work, he sent me to Mt. Tabor school in St John. That was the same school I attended as a young pupil. I worked there for just under a year. While there, I responded

to a request I heard on the local radio (rediffusion) to go to the UK and train as a Psychiatric Nurse. I immediately applied and was successful. I did my training in Stafford and then went to Epsom to do General Nurse Training. Following that I undertook Social Work training and worked as a Social Worker until I retired a few years ago. I enjoy being a member of B.O.N.A, partaking in the Sponsored Walk each year, lending a hand with the annual thanksgiving service, youth seminars and general fundraising activities.

Ceifred R, Goodman

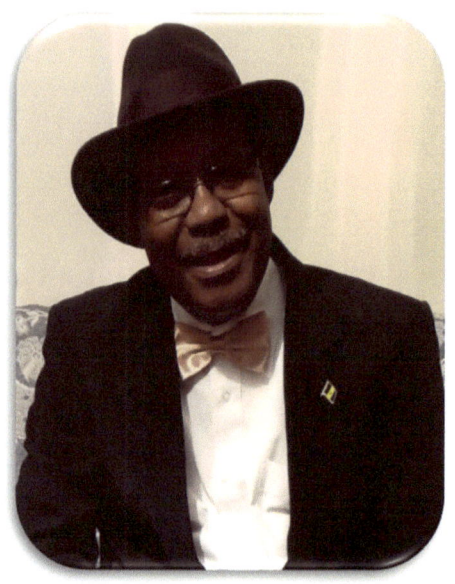

My connection with Barbados Overseas Nurses Association (B.O.N.A) started when I accompanied my late wife (Yvonne Goodman), who was an active Member for many years, I hasten to add. I attended many of the Social Evenings and other Fundraising functions before becoming an Associate Member – as with many other husbands and male partners who were not nurses. Personally, I thought we were only permitted as members simply to do the lifting and carrying. However, we enjoyed it and for that reason I am still a full member. Since then, I have always offered my services to B.O.N.A. I was elected as secretary to B.O.N.A from 2014 to the present time. As Secretary, in addition to taking Minutes and keeping Members updated with the activities of the group and other member organisations, I am responsible for all the graphics, adverts for dances, concerts and booklets for the annual Thanksgiving Service. I liaise regularly with the coordinators of the various committees and assist wherever possible. The organisation aims to maintain an active and healthy lifestyle and encourages others to do likewise.

With that in mind, I took control of the weekly Line Dancing when the former teacher left us high and dry because of a drop in number. Subsequently, there has been a phenomenal growth in numbers (30 +). The social Co-Ordinator, Harold, also holds exercise classes in addition to taking charge of the Line-dancing when I am not available. These joint sessions every Wednesday, run concurrently. Another activity I introduced is the Art classes, using my knowledge and experience to teach others the pleasure of painting and creating their own masterpieces. Not only are these sessions beneficial in terms of fund raising, they also enhance the wellbeing of the members, who look forward to attending each week. We also celebrate birthdays usually with a cake and the happy birthday song.

The atmosphere on Wednesdays is electric and tremendously encouraging.

My other contribution is to the Choir, adding my voice, together with Colvin, to the other melodious voices as the bass duo. And I often sing solos at the Christmas Carols and Nine Lessons. I also take part in the annual fundraising walk.

Margaret Morris-Springer

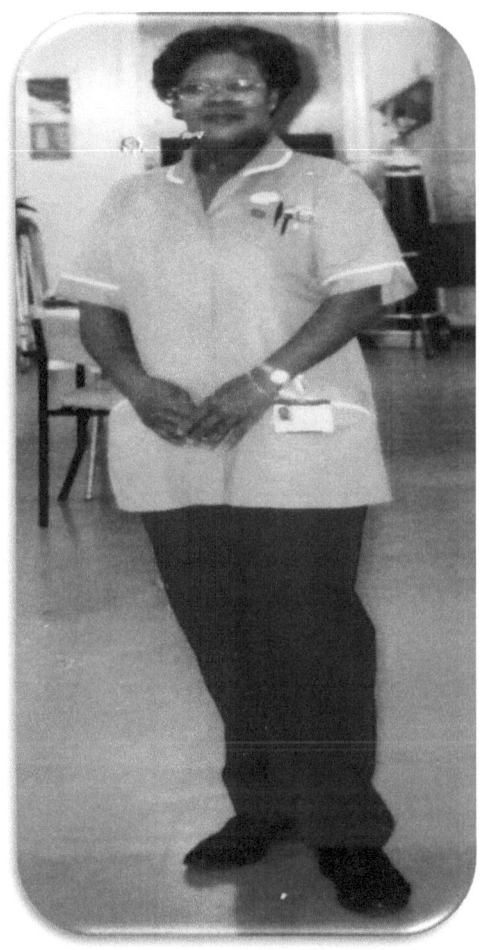

As Vice President of this wonderful Association it is not without admiration and a great feeling of pride, that I wish to congratulate B.O.N.A on their 25 years. The President Mrs Shermane Peters, members past and present, must be immensely proud and I thank them for their sterling work, as we all mark this special occasion.

B.O.N.A has been raising funds for various charities- supporting members and their families when needed. It also gives members a chance to socialise and to meet fellow Barbadians. How the years have flown by, I have held various positions from welfare co-ordinator, social co-ordinator-Assistant, Assistant Treasurer and now Vice President. Thanking all members for their support. To "God be the glory" that he will continue to bless B.O.N.A [UK] and keep the organisation going for years to come.

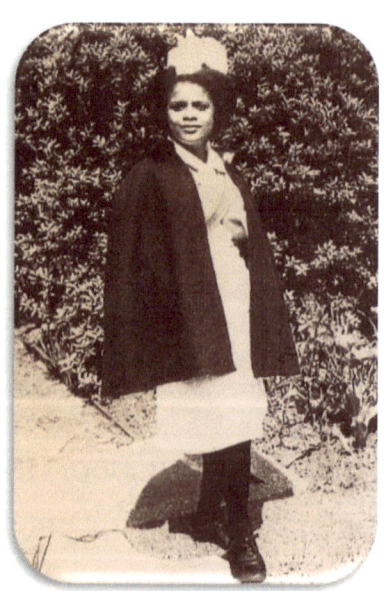

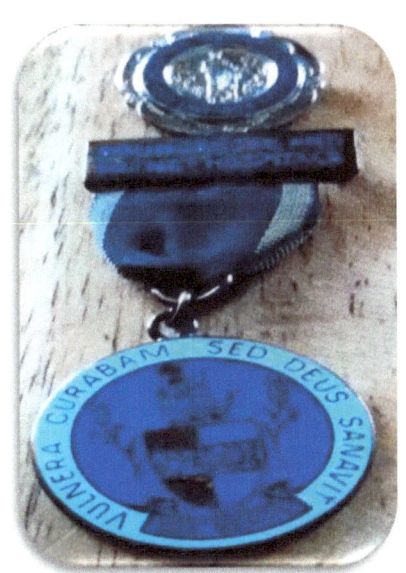

Maria Layne-springer

My name is Maria Layne-Springer (Nee Norville). I came to England on December 15th. 1966 to start my SRN training and worked as a nurse from 1967 – 1983.

Four of us on the flight from Barbados went to the Putney and Bolingbroke Hospital Group. We remained friends even though one of the girls from the group went back to Barbados soon after finishing her training.

The training was uneventful. We did general surgery at Putney and Bolingbroke Hospital, and geriatric at St. John's Hospital and orthopaedics at Battersea. All these hospitals are now closed!

After completing my SRN Training which I got in 1971, I did a six-month Post Graduation Course of male surgery and genito-urinary nursing at West Middlesex Hospital.

From there, I went to Moorfield Eye Hospital to train as an eye nurse. I had no real interest in midwifery. I was already aware of Moorfields' as I started my nurse training in Barbados. The Sister-in charge of the Eye Unit in Barbados was trained at Moorfields and worked there, really enjoyed the experience. Also, when I was changing Wards, Sister told me if I was ever stuck for a speciality, I should choose eyes. While at Moorfields, I moved to Croydon and worked on the Eye Unit at St. Georges' Hospital, then went to Waddon Hospital in Croydon.

A word about Waddon Hospital:

This hospital was built in 1896 for treating infectious diseases, and later treated patients with tuberculosis. In 1930, an operating theatre was added. The hospital then became a geriatric unit, along with patients needing eye surgical operations from the Mayday branch of Moorfields Hospital. Waddon closed in 1984 and now nothing remains of the hospital. The site is now part of Valley Park, an out-of-town shopping centre, containing a variety of shops, restaurants, and an Ikea store.

I went to Waddon in 1976 and worked there until I resigned 1983. Like many surgical advances at that time, contact lenses were the "in thing" in eye care.

My contribution was to test early lenses for ease of wear, application and removal and the length of time there could be worn before becoming uncomfortable.

At first, they covered most of the front of the eye (haptic lenses) until they reach the soft gels that we now have.

I thoroughly enjoyed my work in the NHS and only gave it up as my circumstances changed. Of course, there were difficult patches, but I believe with time and patience we can overcome most obstacles that come our way as we work to make meaningful contributions to the societies in which we live.

Angela Alleyne

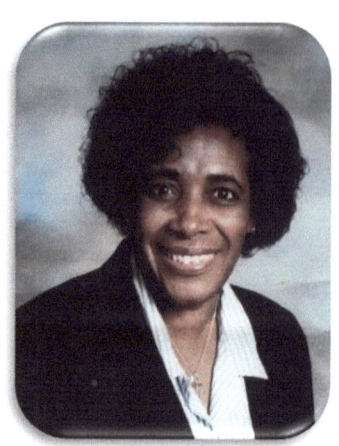

I was born in Barbados and went to school at both St. Pauls School and the Parkinson School. The early death of my mother when I was nine years old had a great impact on my siblings and I consequently grew up with my cousins.

In my late teens, I decided to leave the Island. At that time, the UK was recruiting young people to train and work for the NHS as nurses, and staff for London Transport. At nineteen years old, I was on the plane travelling to the UK to qualify as a nurse. My nursing career has been varied. I continued studying after completing my Enrolled Nurses Training. To complete my state registration, Midwifery, and orthopaedic Nursing certificates. After six years in the UK, I returned to Barbados to work as a registered nurse for a short period. After one year I returned to England.

After completing my Midwifery, I worked as an agency staff nurse at Mount Vernon Burns Unit and was promoted to ward sister in 1975. I met my husband when working at Mount Vernon, then came marriage and children. After the birth of my first child, I took a break from nursing before returning to work as a part time staff nurse.

I have worked hard but the social scene in London during the late sixties and early seventies greatly compensated for the hard work. There were house parties and night clubs; there were times we would get in on a

Sunday morning minutes before our shifts was due to start after a Saturday night out! On other occasions, we would be lounging around in the nurses' home on our days off reminiscing with fellow Barbadians and nurses of different nationalities.

I remembered when two other Barbadians nurses and I bought a pig head and decided to make some 'Bajan souse' – a delicacy from the Caribbean- late one evening. We put the pigs head on to cook, and while it was cooking, we went to watch TV. We became so engrossed in an Alfred Hitchcock film that we completely forgot about the pig's head sizzling away in the saucepan producing more white smoke with no water left.

My nursing experience and skills have been useful in family life. One of my daughters had to wear a corrective "plaster jacket" for an extended period, and another child was seriously injured in road traffic accident. My caring for them prevented further complications and allowed recovery treatment at home. Outside of nursing, I took an active interest in my children's education from the early years until university. I was also a member of the parent-teachers association becoming chairperson, I was also a Parent -Governor for many years at their first and middle school.

It was at times hectic, while still working but a great learning and rewarding experience. I helped to prevent accidents small and large, involving school, children, and parents from escalating further, to assisting children in improving confidence by reading with them. All my children are university graduates.

I like the diversity of life in England. After five years of residence in England, I applied for and got a British Passport. Despite problems with racism and housing, living in England has been a wealth of knowledge, learning and travel. I have met people of many different nationalities. When I return to Barbados, I like catching up with family and friends. My favourite past time is early mornings on the beach. I am currently a Member of Barbados Overseas Nurses Association, the Sickle Cell Society, and the NHS Retirement Fellowship. Well done to B.O.N.A for reaching 25 years.

UK "Bajan nurses" together with homeland "Bajan nurses" during the millennium celebration in Barbados 2000

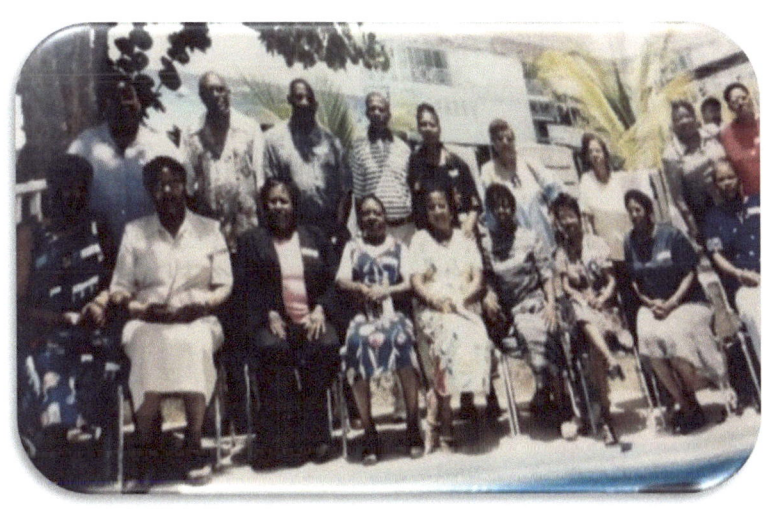

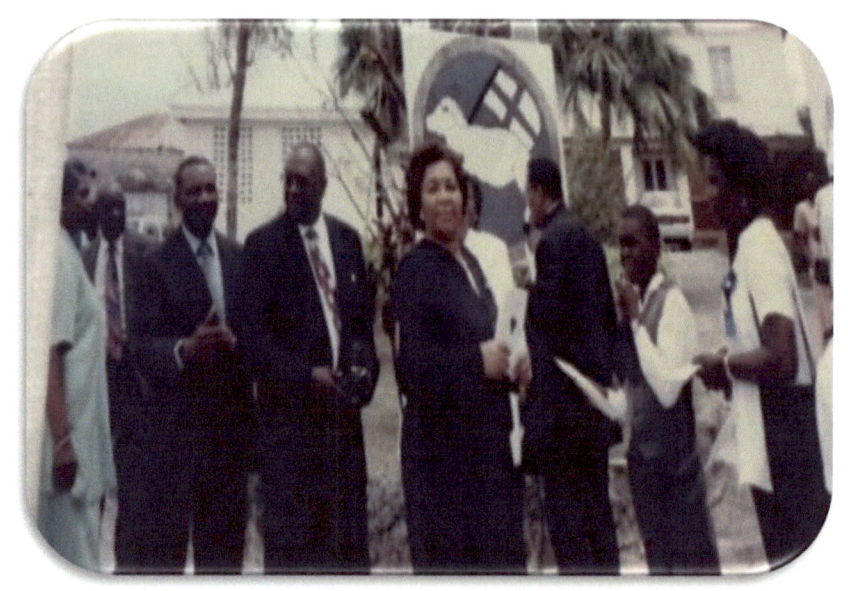

Nurses and Friends 2000

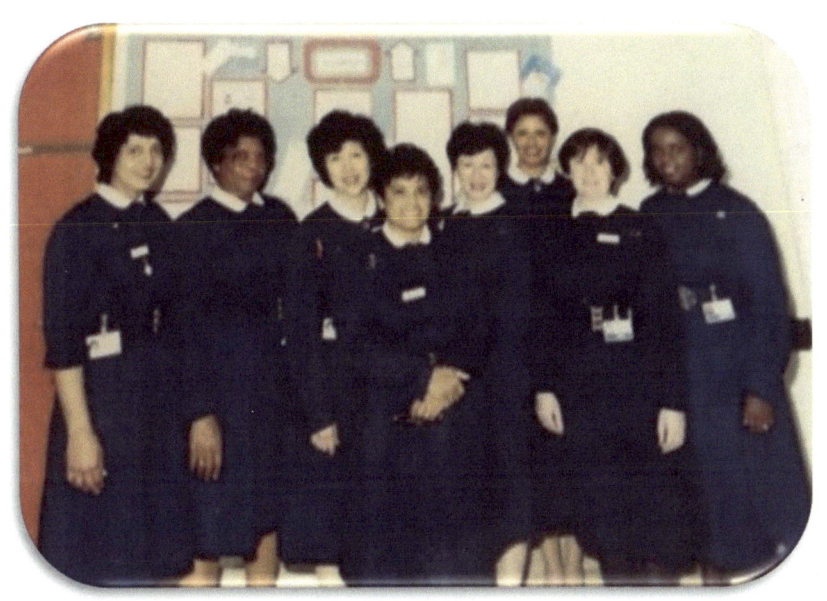

Barbara with nursing colleagues

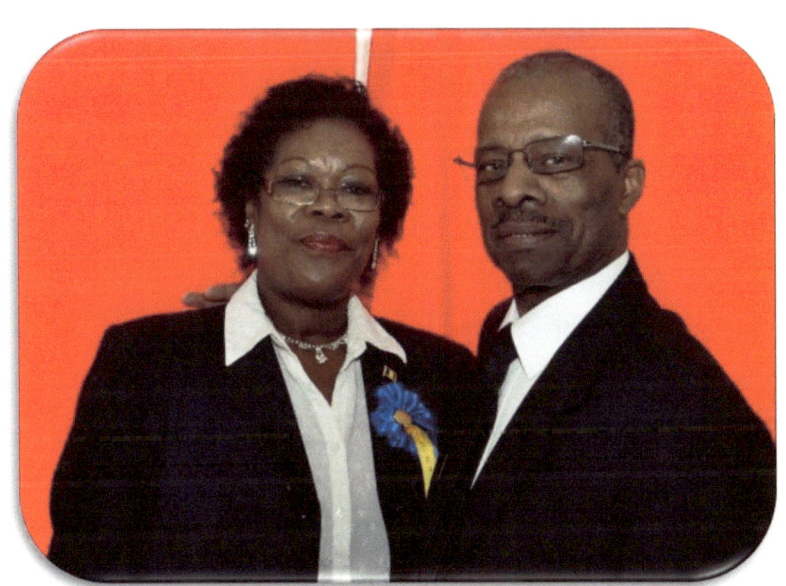

Margaret & Colvin

Shirley Clarke

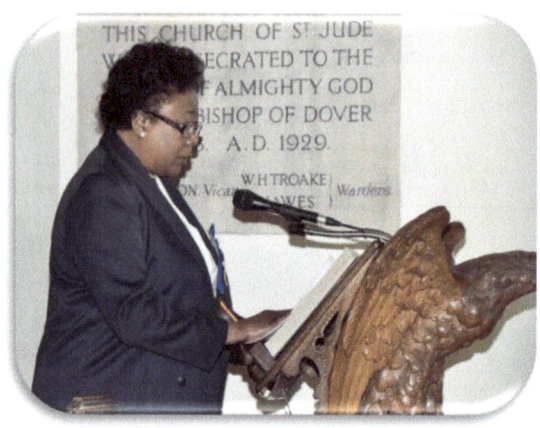

When I arrived in the UK, I started my NHS training at Queen Victoria, East Grinstead, then Plastic Surgery and Burns. I then studied at Pembury Hospital RGN, and to St. Thomas's Hospital in Churchy Intensive Care.

I joined the organisation after I left the NHS and congratulate B.O.N.A on reaching twenty-five (25) years of service of giving back to the community, both in the UK and especially to the deserving causes in Barbados and elsewhere. B.O.N.A also have been a source of keeping in touch with others of the same profession, keeping up to date, socialising and taking part with the various activities of the association, mixing with other liked organisations and making new friends, building meaningful relationships.

Waple's Story
My Journey within the NHS UK

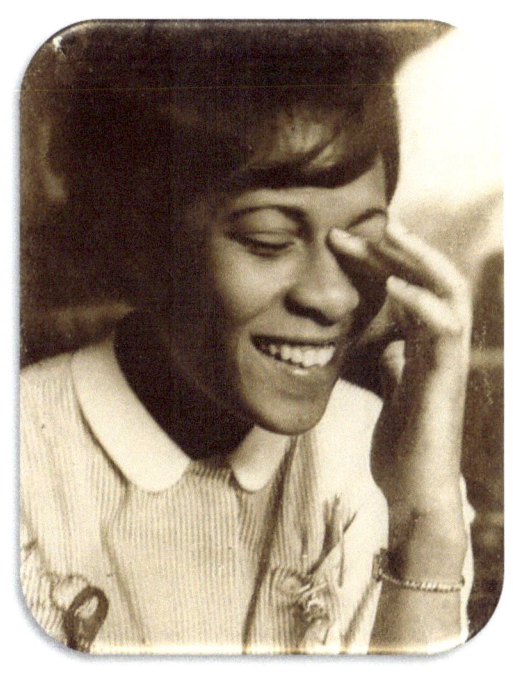

I was nineteen years old when I arrived in the UK in October 1968 to begin my nurse training. It was my first experience of travelling abroad and I was a little apprehensive as I was travelling alone. A representative from the Barbados High Commission met me at Heathrow
Airport and gave me instructions for my train journey to Waterloo Station and my onward journey to the Southampton Group Hospitals.
I arrived at the Hospital on a wet, cold, and grey day, one week before my nurse training was due to start. I was directed to work on the geriatric ward prior to

starting my training. My first experience of nursing was being handed a bowl of water and told to wash a very obese female. I instantly felt panicky and scared and thought to myself 'what an introduction to nursing'!

Working and studying at the same time was challenging. However, I made many friends which made the experience both enjoyable and rewarding. Plus, there were always new things to learn and practice.

Receiving my first pay packet was quite a surprise. I had expected a higher wage for my hard work, but the wages were small and did not go far. After I had sent money home to repay the cost of my flight to the UK, there was extraordinarily little left for me to save or spend.

Having completed my general nursing training, I decided to pursue other nursing courses to broaden my knowledge and gain further qualifications. First, I embarked on a course in thoracic nursing. I then studied to become a State Certified Midwife, Family Planning Nurse and Practice Nurse.

During my career, I worked at several hospitals in London,

Carlma De Abreau

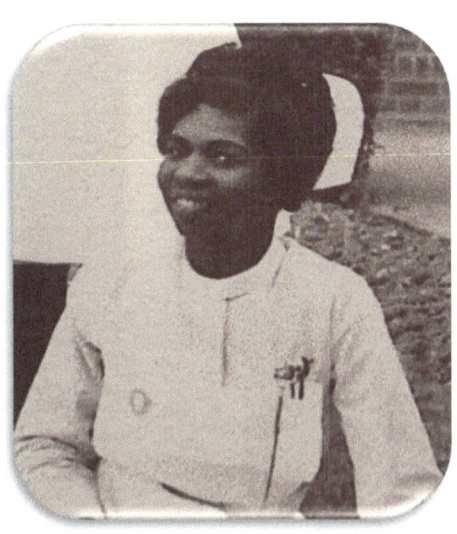

I was one of the Founder Members of this great organisation, the Barbados Overseas Nurses Association. Although I did not reach the pristine heights of President, I feel very proud that my younger sister has attained that position, wishing her and all the Members of B.O.N.A much success in the good work they are doing. My story began when, at the tender age of eighteen (18), I embarked on a journey to this "green and pleasant land" to study

nursing. I trained in Essex at St Georges Hospital and Old Church Hospital as a General Nurse, gaining my State Registered Nurse Certificate. My employment in the NHS included Queen Mary's Hospital in Carshalton, Mayday Hospital in Croydon as a Theatre nurse which led me to specialise in Theatre Nursing. I finally retired as a Senior Theatre Manager at St. Thomas's Hospital in London. Through it all, I married and have son, a Graduate Engineer.

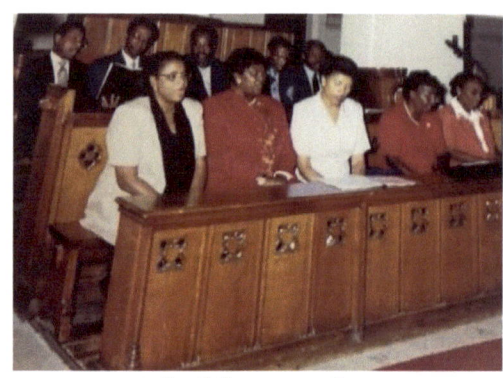

(Pictures provided by Barbara Brewster MBE)

including The Middlesex Hospital, Brompton Hospital and Kings College Hospital. I also worked as a midwife in a private sector hospital.

After I got married and had children, I decided to work part-time so that I could spend more time with my family. When my children started school, I extended my working hours. I spent the last 25 years of my career as a Practice Nurse and Family Planning Nurse Specialist. I have had mostly positive experiences during my nursing career. I have had the privilege of caring for my patients and making a difference to their lives. I feel that I have achieved my goal which was to make a positive contribution to the British National Health Service.

I am now retired; I am grateful to God that He graciously gave me the opportunity to fulfil the dream and ambition I fostered so many years ago as a teenager in Barbados.

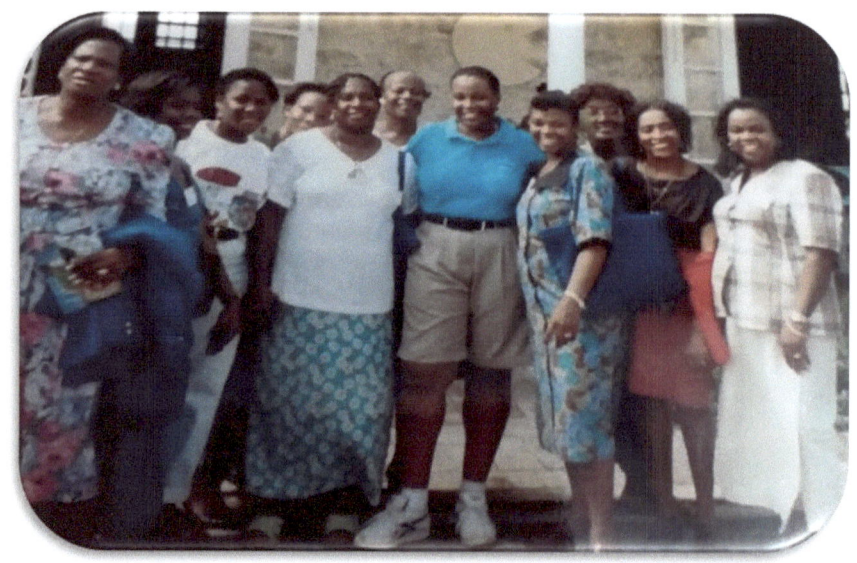

Members of B.O.N.A Celebrating the century (2000) with nursing professionals and friends in Barbados

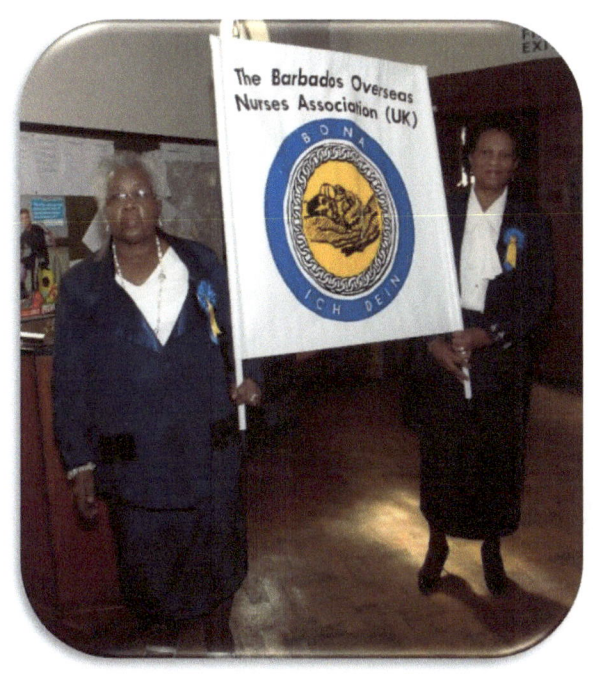

Thelma Walcott & Waple Baird
Flag Bearers 2011 Thanksgiving Service

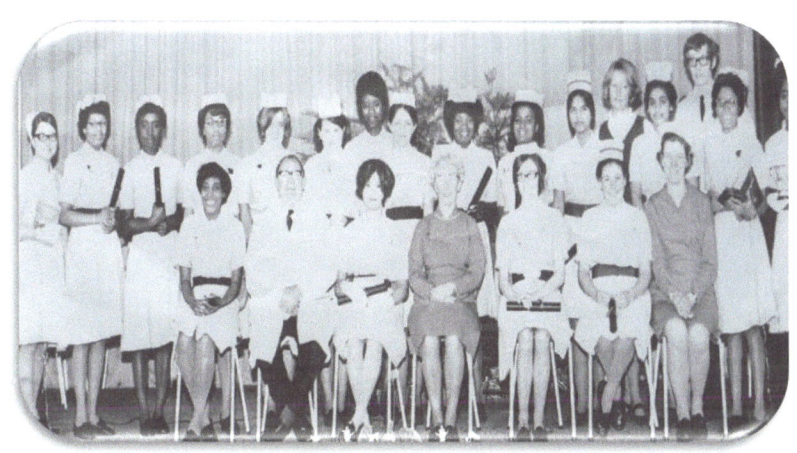

Spot the Bajan Nurses in this group

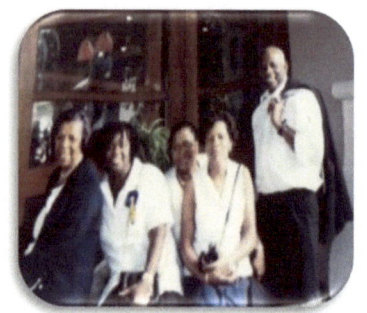 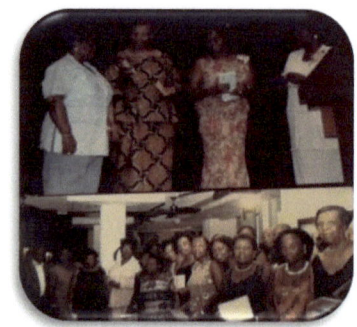

Lorraine Whitehall's Journey in the NHS

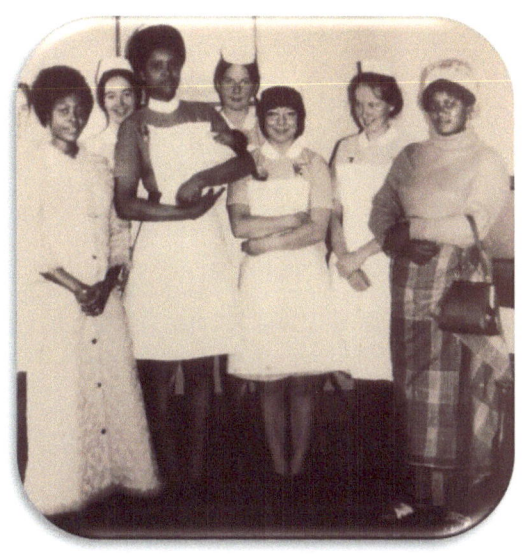

My journey in the NHS started in 1963 when I had not long turned eighteen years of age and got the chance to obtain a place on the nurses recruitment scheme which was set up in Barbados by the British Government and co-ordinated by a lady known as MS Griffiths, whose office was situated at Fontabelle, Herbert House, St Michael.

Ms Griffiths dealt with all the formalities necessary prior to persons being recruited to the UK for example: interview by herself, arranging a medical check at Enmore Heath Centre and a basic English exam. I managed to be accepted and arrived in the

UK on March 27th, 1963 and was in Lincolnshire, please see below, details of my journey in the NHS.

1. Branston Hall Hospital-Main hospital for a 2-year course Congland Hall Hospital, Gainsborough- Seconded here. St Georges Hospital, Lincoln City seconded here, qualified as an S.E.N further and went back to Branston hospital to work in that capacity until in 1966 to pursue further training to gain S.R.N. qualification.

2. St. Albans city Hospital, Herts- Gained S.R.N qualification here and then worked as a staff Nurse on our Private Wing for about a year before leaving to pursue Midwifery training. I missed St Albans a lot.

3. Perivale Maternity Hospital, Greenford where I obtained my part one Certificate of Midwifery.

4. Queen Elizabeth II Hospital Luton Beds. I gained part 2 Midwifery, Luton/Dunstable Hospital.

Weir Maternity Hospital -Started here as a staff midwife in 1972 but later re located to St. Georges Tooting.

In 1973 Promoted to Midwifery Sister at St. Georges in 1974 Where I stayed until my retirement. My son, only child, was born at St George's Hospital. I was

extremely well looked after by the team whom I had worked with for some years. After 31 years, A very splendid retirement party was held for me and I absolutely enjoyed the occasion.
I absolutely enjoyed the Midwifery too. Even to this day, I still meet most of the mums whom I cared for, but I do not always remember all of them, however, one had to remain polite and receptive on these occasions.

I thank our heavenly father for all my Professional Achievements and pray for satisfactory progressive long-term career paths for all those who remain in the NHS. At present. Those joining may God bless, always guide, and inspire them all. Amen.

Marie Greenidge *nee Belgrave*
My journey to the "Mother Country"

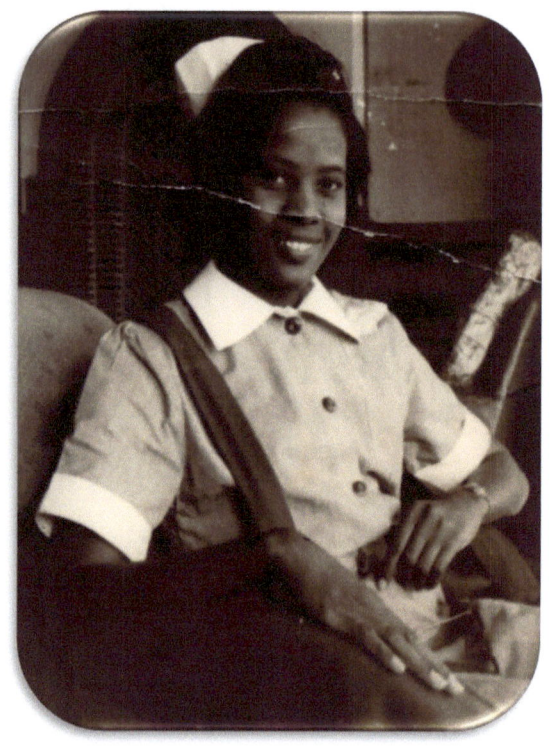

After I met the criteria for Nurse training in the UK via the Nursing selection committee of Barbados, I left Barbados at the end of December 1961 from the then known Seawell Airport, aboard the Caledonian Airways: a Scottish charter airline which ceased operations early 1970's. I still have the carbon copy stub of my airline ticket.

Although a journey to the unknown, it was an exciting venture. During the first leg of the journey there was some problem with the plane, we landed at the Azores evidently to have the problem fixed. I remember it being very hot and humid, four of us moved together, we were very thirsty - decided to purchase cold drinks which we started to drink as soon as they were presented, between us we only had UK currency which the attendant had no idea of any exchange rate or never seen this

currency before, as a result it ended with laughter and us having free drinks.

For the second leg of the journey the plane could not land at Gatwick due to adverse weather conditions, this was now January 1962 and recorded as the big freeze and one of the coldest winters on record. The

flight was diverted to Shannon Airport and then to Bournemouth, after overnight stay at a gloriously warm Hotel, we were transported by Coach to the main line station, we were greeted by an official from The Barbados embassy before boarding the train on our way to Leicester. We were met and transported by Hospital minibus to Markfield Hospital. This was a challenging experience, getting used to icicles, snow and the dark mornings, believing that it was still sleeping time instead of reporting for the induction session, however, I gradually came to terms with the new way of life and the four seasons. My annual salary was £299.00 for the first Year then £315.00 for the second Year from that £128.00 went towards Board and lodging plus 6% monthly towards Superannuation, like most of us of that period, we had to repay the loan from the Barbados Government.

At the end of my second Year I moved to London to commence General Nurse training at Mile End Hospital, later moved from the area got married and started a family, during which time I have worked all hours (as the saying goes) in the private sector, before re-joining the NHS. I commenced working at May Day Hospital towards the end of 1990.

I was introduced to B.O.N.A by the late Pearleen Harris by letter which was then the more general mode of communication. I joined the Association in 1994 during its first year of inception. I can also remember the first fund raising Christmas social held that Year which raised just over £300.00, this prompted the founder members to open an account with Barclay's Bank Thornton Heath. During my membership I have taken on the role of Secretary which I held for eight years. I have always been willing to help as needed, especially with social

fundraising events, and in keeping with the aims and objectives of the Association: To assist those less fortunate than ourselves, both in the UK and Barbados.

I would like to end by adding my sincere congratulations to B.O.N.A on reaching its Silver Anniversary.

"Coming to Britain" Monica Gordon

In 1965 I decided to come to Britain to train as a nurse. It was daunting and challenging as I had never left home before. After all the planning, of us set off and ended up at the same hospital. I did two years training. It was long hours and awfully hard work. Lots of lifting. I was able to gain the knowledge and skills and confidence which allowed me to make a living working and contributing to the National Health Service for many years. It also enabled me to travel to different countries to visit Family or to go sightseeing. Some of the interesting places we visited were the Dominican Republic. Jamaica, Cuba, Italy, Malta, Guernsey, Jersey. Cruise to the Caribbean, cruise to the Panama Canal. I was able to go to La Gomera in the Canary Isles to see my brother, Philip, and his friend Randal set sail on an epic voyage, rowing 3000 miles across the Atlantic Ocean to Barbados. It was amazing, and an awe inspiring and lasting memory.

I became a member of B.O.N.A ten years ago and became continually active in taking part in all the fundraising event, especially the annual sponsored walk. However, due to recent ill health, I was unable to take in the last walk.

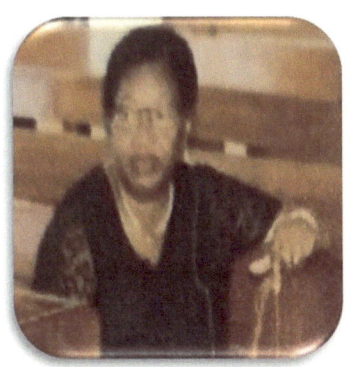

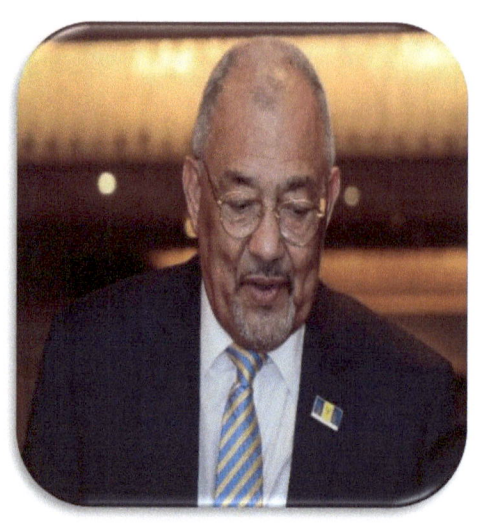

Harold Springer

I was born in Barbados in 1940, I immigrated to the U.K in 1961. It was a cold grey April day when I arrived; it was night-time, so I was unable to see a lot. Next morning, I was up bright and early. I wanted to see this place we all called our "Mother Country". The others were still asleep, this was about 7.00 in the morning. Everything was still quiet I peeped out - to my surprise seven o`clock – no sun. If I were in Barbados, I would have milked the cow and taken the sheep out. About eight or nine o`clock there was some movement. My cousin and his girlfriend began to make a movement. They said to me that people in England do not get up that early on weekends!

At the weekend I decided to visit my uncle who lived near Regents Park, he came to get me. We had to travel by Underground, the Northern line, we travelled to the Oval tube station, went down to the platform. When I got there the smell from trains went straight up my nostrils! While waiting I saw something moving between the rails, I had a good look and realised it was a mouse, it was dark grey in colour it was the first time I had seen mice that colour. We reached Regents Park.

But the smell from the underground still lingered in my nostrils, I decided to put my finger up my nostril to help get rid of the smell, to my surprise the finger came out the same colour as the mouse.

I joined B.O.N.A. on the 20.5.13, before becoming a member I supported the Organisation going to their dances and other functions. It was at one of these dances at Brixton Town Hall I met my wife so I decided I would give something back to the community.

I officially became a member on the 20.5.13. After joining I would help organize some events I was asked if I wanted to be part of the many committees which form the Organisation. I thought about the Education Committee but decided to join the Social Committee.

This Committee organises social events: dances, post valentine events, concerts where the money raised from these events go to B.O.N.A to help other charities here and in the Caribbean. The Social Committee Members also provide food, drinks, cakes, sweetbread, fish cakes where the donations raised are added to help the fundraising.

After joining the social Committee, I decided to take a more active role. When our line dancing instructor left and Ceifred agreed he would take over the role of dancing instructor, he introduced music to dance to reggae, soca, soul and not just your regular country and western music. The group started to grow from our usual ten or twelve, now it is between twenty to thirty and is still growing.

Ceifred decided as the group was growing, he would find out if any of the group was interested in other activities. One day after line dancing, he said if any were interested in art, he would be willing to teach us. A few of us decided we would like to have a try, he told us what we needed, the next week after line dancing, we gathered around a table.

I was a complete novice to art. I am an incredibly determined person and do not like to fail. My first attempt was to sketch a glass vase, my attempt was quite good. Since then I have continued with my painting, this has added a new chapter to my life, thanks to Ceifred and B.O.N.A.

A few years after joining the Social Committee I was asked if I would like to take over the role of Social Coordinator as the President was wearing two hats being and President and the Social Coordinator. At first, I was not quite sure but decided to have a go as I said earlier, I don`t like being a failure.

At present I am still doing the job I am still learning. Since taking over the Social Committee Coordinator`s role I had an accident and had to have a hip replacement. After my operation I had to do a lot of exercises to help rebuild the muscle in my hip and thigh. I enjoyed doing these exercises, kept close to the Physio and learned the routines, now I use them to take the line dancers through a warm-up session before the line dancing starts.

Gloria Gittens
My Journey through the NHS and B.O.N.A

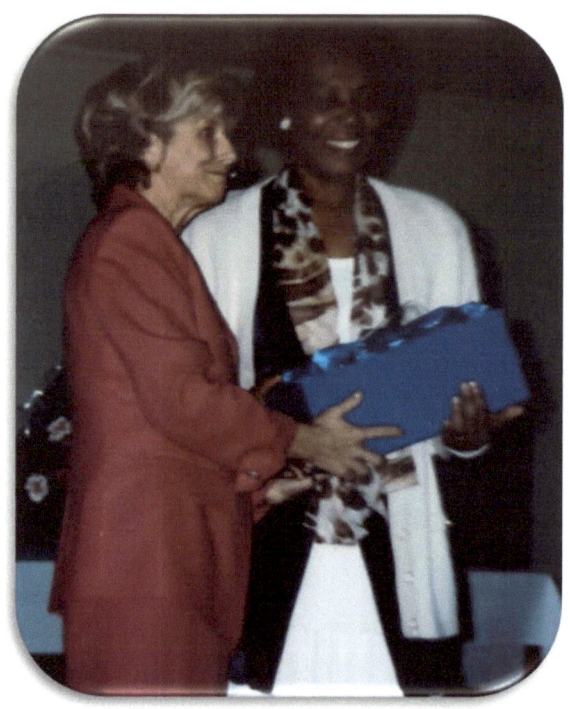

After completing my training, I worked as a Health Care Assistant in the NHS for many years, receiving a valuable and well-earned Long Service Recognition award when I retired. I joined the Barbados Overseas Nurses Association (B.O.N.A) in 2004 and after my retirement, I was able to be a more active member, getting involved in many of the activities of the organisation.

I am active member of the Social Committee, Care and Support and I love singing in the Choir. I have also contributed to the planning of the Annual Thanksgiving Service especially the 25-year celebration service where I was incredibly happy to read one of the lessons.

I always enjoy all the social aspects of the organisation, including the annual sponsored walks, the concerts, Dinner & Dances, Christmas Lunch, lunch Cruises, the weekly exercises, the line dancing lessons, all adding to our fundraising efforts.

I have had positive feedback from members who are at present unable to attend regular meetings, but still offer support whenever they can. May God bless B.O.N.A and its Members as they continue to grow in excellence.

Carmita Neblett
My Journey in the NHS and B.O.N.A

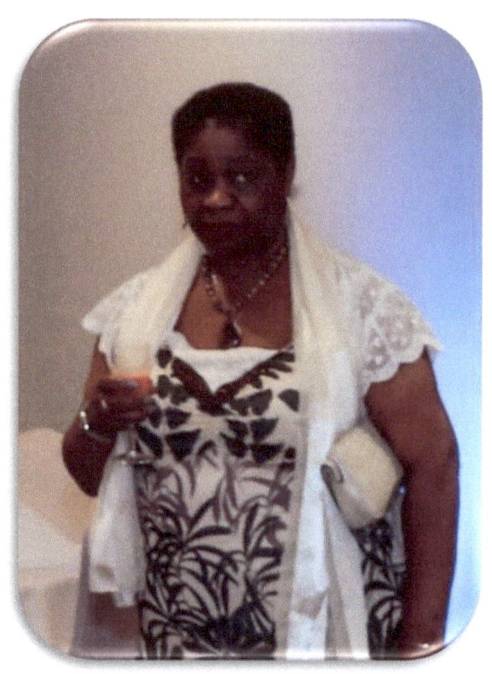

I joined Barbados Overseas Nurses Association in 2018. I was introduced by my friend Gloria Gittens. I met up with and she is very friendly. I look forward to meeting up when we have our monthly meetings. I also enjoy helping in the many fundraising events during the year. I am a member of the choir, taking part in the singing at concerts and church services. Every Wednesday we have line-dancing and exercise which I enjoy very much. B.O.N.A. is a terribly busy organisation, and now that I am retired, I can offer my services by getting more involved in all the social activities, including the art classes. This year I hope my Art will be featured in the Annual Calendar for 2020.

Although I have not been a member for 25 years, I can see the benefits of being a member of this association so much that I introduced my brother. He also enjoys the activities and gets involved with the events. My Blessings.

Golda Griffiths

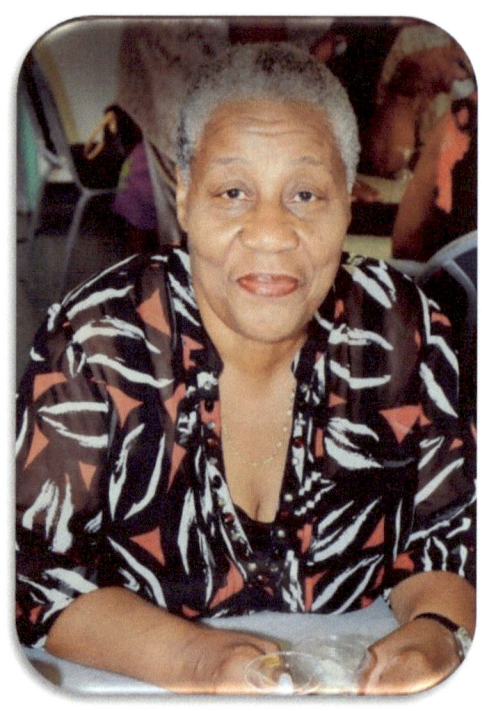

My Journey in the NHS and B.O.N.A

I arrived in England on the May 1964 at Heathrow Airport on our journey to Victoria station we saw the changing of the guards.

We travelled from Victoria station to Haywards Heath West Sussex and was met by the assistant Matron of Pouch lands Hospital, which was a mental hospital and not a general hospital. I stayed there a year and went on to Southwestern where I trained as a state Enrolled Nurse. I worked in several hospitals, Sunderland Maternity hospital,

Westminster Hospital, South London, Croydon General, and finally Mayday hospital where I trained as a Registered Nurse and worked on the Gastroenterology ward until my retirement.

Now that I am retired, I am a member of B.O.N.A. and offer my services to this busy Organisation. I am pleased that it has reached its 25th year and that I am part of its Growth.

Revd Jackie Cockfield
My Journey in the NHS and B.O.N.A

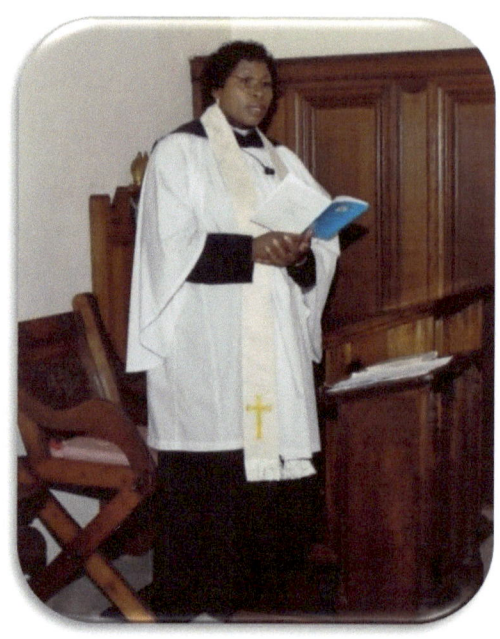

After training as a nurse, I worked and remained in the intensive care Nursing setting until my retirement. Firstly, I joined the staff in the General Intensive Care Unit at St. Georges Hospital, Tooting. A few years passed, and I then transferred to the Intensive Care Unit within the same hospital. Following gradual promotion, I became a senior Sister with a staff numbering seventy-two in total. Along the way I was encouraged by members of the clergy and others who felt and apparently could see that I had a ministerial calling. I was not aware of this calling myself, or subconsciously, did I choose to ignore!! I thought, no, cannot possibly be me and tried to avoid any conversations or engage any thoughts pertaining to the matter for as long as I could. However, my stubbornness gave way to acceptance.

Following studies and training, I was ordained to the priesthood in the Church of England in 2009. I am the Assistant Priest at Mitcham Parish Church, non-Stipendiary appt which means I am not paid; my services are voluntary.

This goes to show that God has a plan for each of us and always catches up with us in the end, despite our excuses. My academic qualifications include: Intensive Care Nursing Diploma; BA (Hons.) Ministerial Theology; BA (Hons) Social Science.

Jean Millar

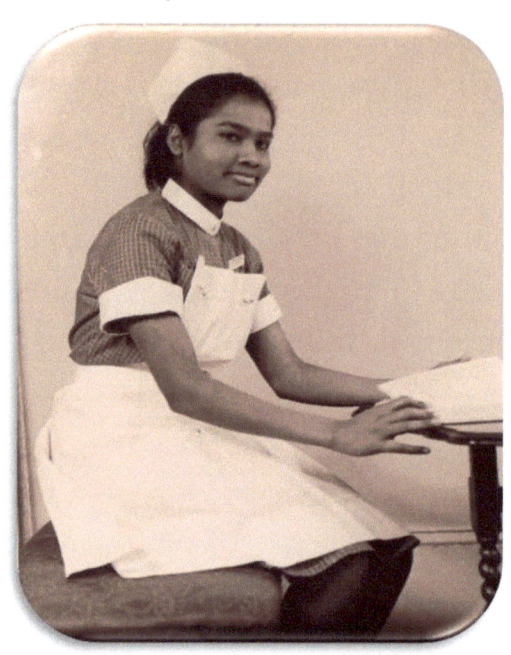

My Journey in the NHS and B.O.N.A

I left Trinidad aboard a cruise ship, "The Northern Star", on September 4th. 1966 to study nursing in the United Kingdom. I shared a cabin with three other passengers, and arrived at Southampton 11 days later, then took the boat train to Victoria Station. The three passengers who shared the cabin left for Yorkshire. I was met by a member from the British Council who then escorted me to Grove Park Hospital where I completed a two-year training in Chest diseases. I qualified as a State Enrolled nurse in 1968.

Following qualifications, I moved to Long grove Hospital to do my Student nurse Training,

Once qualified as a Registered Mental Nurse, then left for St. Charles Hospital to do further training in General Nursing and qualified as Registered General Nurse.

I returned to Psychiatry and worked at tooting Bec Hospital south Western and lastly worked in an assessment Ward unit at St. Thomas Hospital for the elderly, mentored both student nurses and Health Care Assistants especially those completing the National Vocational Qualification in Care. The NVQ trainees went on to complete both courses now a fully fledge trained nurses. There was a lot of movements between patients and staff within the Unit. I retired in 2006 and joined B.O.N.A a little later and participated in the group work in arts. Mr C Goodman being the Educator thereby developing my skills in painting with some of the work going to produce calendars. I enjoy all the activities such as line dancing, concerts etc. In closing, I wish the organisation and my member-colleagues happy 25th Anniversary and long may we continue to do so.

Isalene Carter

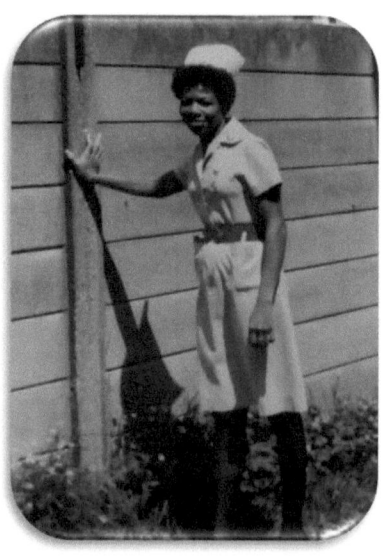

I left Barbados on the 4th October 1969 to pursue a career in Nursing, and I commenced my SEN training soon after arriving in the UK. On completion, I, unfortunately had trouble trying to secure a place to do my SRN training. I did Ophthalmic Nursing training, immediately on completion of that course, I was finally accepted to do my SRN, followed by my SCM. I continued to work in the NHS in various areas such as the Intensive Care and Coronary Care, as a newly qualified nurse. Those areas could be a bit scary at first, but one soon gained confidence and functioned efficiently. I also managed a large outpatient's department.

Finally, I was appointed as a ward sister on an Orthopaedic ward, which was very stressful at times, especially during the winter months with the shortage of staff and beds, but I had a very supportive staff, and enjoyed those years.

I joined B.O.N.A in 1994, served on the Executive and Social committee. I also held other positions, including assistant Secretary and assistant Treasurer. I am now retired and relocated back in Barbados. I make annual visits to the UK, during time I willingly offer my assistance at various functions of the organisation.

Cecelia Rodrigues

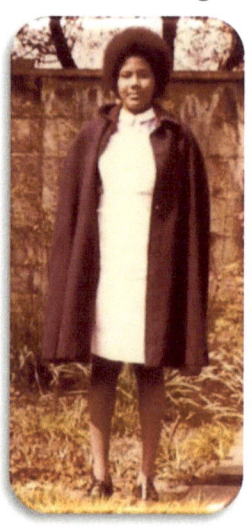

I was recruited from Grenada, a British Colony to start a career in the UK. I came to England aged 18, in 1974. My first nursing experience was at Lewisham General where I completed my SRN training. I later moved to the West Midlands and worked at various hospitals, moving to a senior role.

Whilst living in the West Midlands, I married and had 2 daughters. I appreciated the opportunities that were available in England and apart from my nursing experience, I took the opportunity to do further studies and gained a degree in Business and Finance. I have now retired and joined the NHS fellowship to which I recruited Shermane Peters, President of BONA. She also recruited me to join BONA. My years in England have been very pleasant in general and successful. I have enjoyed the educational and cultural opportunities available to me. My first couple of years were however negatively tainted by a few individuals who were ignorant of what and who Caribbean people were. I wish BONA all the best for the next 25 years and beyond.

So, congratulations to all past and current members of BONA on your 25th anniversary.
 "Go forward in peace, joy and love."

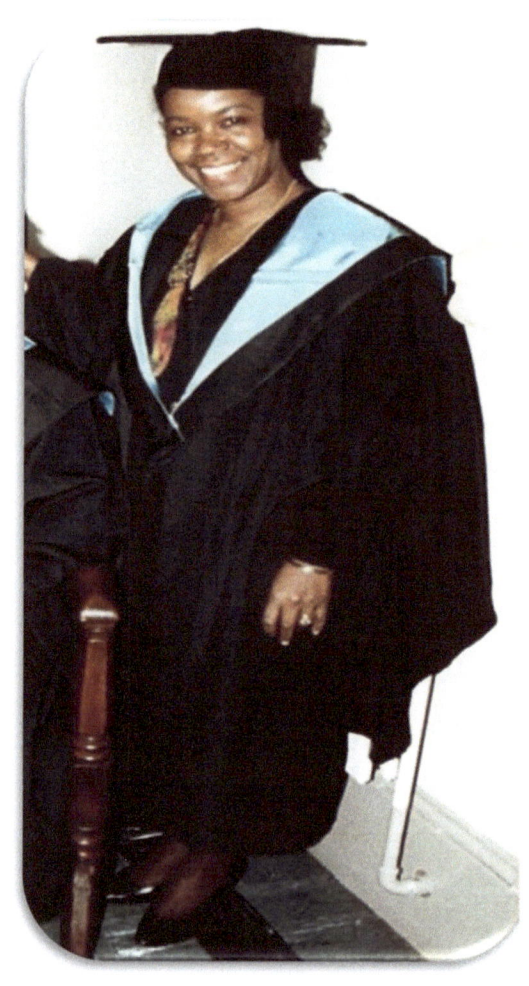

Yvonne Goodman*
My Journey

I came to the UK in 1958 like so many other Bajan young girls to study nursing. I was destined to St. Paul's Hospital in Winchester, Hampshire where I stayed until I sat my exams but did not complete my two years. I came to London, during which time I met and married my husband. I returned to nursing in 1962 when I realised that nursing was my professional calling, and completed my training at St. Benedict's Hospital, Church Lane, Tooting.

Our family moved to East London where I worked at Mile End Hospital for three years before returning to South London. After the birth of my third child, I worked at Putney Hospital until I joined Wandsworth Social Services in 1972.

My nursing qualifications equipped me with the necessary skills I needed in administering medication and traditional nursing care in dealing with people of a vulnerable age. My responsibilities included overseeing a care home with a population of 52 elderly residents, including the provision for respite, and developing a range of services conducive to their wellbeing.

Management of resources included proper maintenance of the building and its facilities, staff management, recruitment of new staff, training, delegation of duties, discipline, budgeting, administration on day to day basis, and coordinating the systems that facilitate the work within the service.

My training as a nurse gave me the knowledge and professional expertise to carry out my duties successfully and deal with any issue facing the residents and staff. In this type of work Elaine, you needed tolerance, ability to listen, counselling, communication skills, assessment, supervision, report writing, organizing, leadership workload, management, and good housekeeping.

Ongoing training was a must if I were to do my job proficiently, especially when working for the Council, so I attended the following courses:
1. Introduction to Social Services 1974
2. Principles & Practice Management W.L.I
3. Management Officer in Charge (OIC) 1978
4. Reality Orientation Seminar 1979
5. Long-term Care 1985
6. Selection Interviewing 1988
7. Certificate in CQSW 1990

After a long membership to B.O.N.A, I became President in 2015 and despite my long illness I was determined to maintain the standards set by previous presidents, and raise the levels of achievements wherever necessary. My vision for the association was to see an increase in membership even for those people outside of nursing, and including our young people who are desperately in need of guidance and direction, helping them to find their way over the obstacles of unconscious bias,

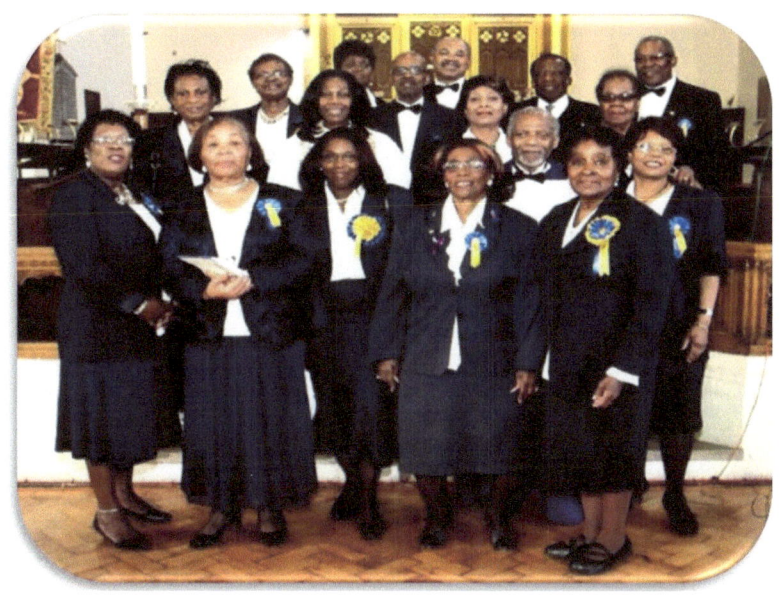

B.O.N.A Choir: Margaret, Waple, Cynthia, Millicent, Shermane, Gloria, Oriel, Colvin, Elkin, Anne, Norma, Gladstone, Hammington, Irma, Elaine, Conchita, Ceifred

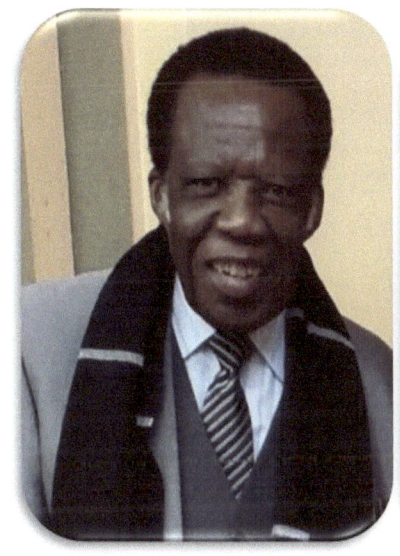

Hammington Marshall
Choir Master

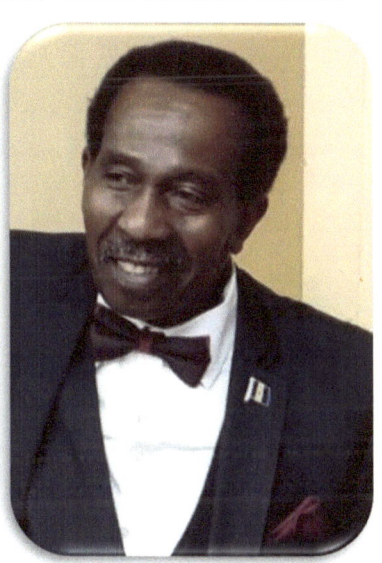

Anderson Seale
Organist

Recipients of our Fundraising efforts

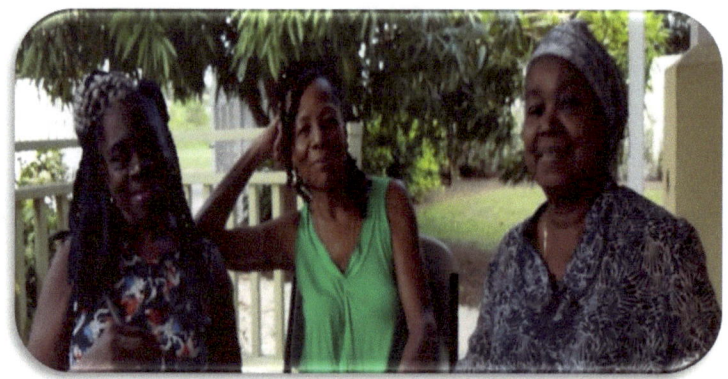

Barbados Kidney Association

(President Yvonne Goodman* & member Isalene Carter of B.O.N.A with Shirley Knight of the Barbados Kidney Association 2016)

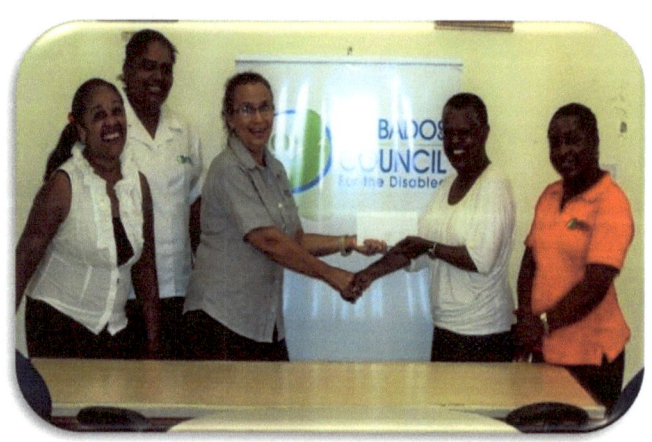

Mrs. Tudor, on behalf of the children with disabilities in Barbados 2013, accepting a cheque from Maria (B.O.N.A) Presentation of a donation

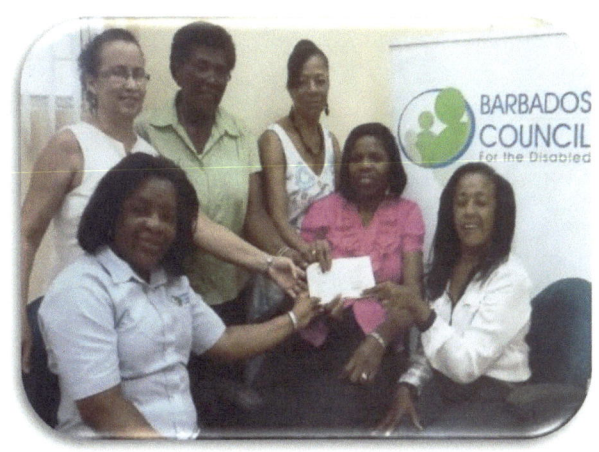

Julia and Isalene presenting a donation to members of the Barbados Council for the Disabled

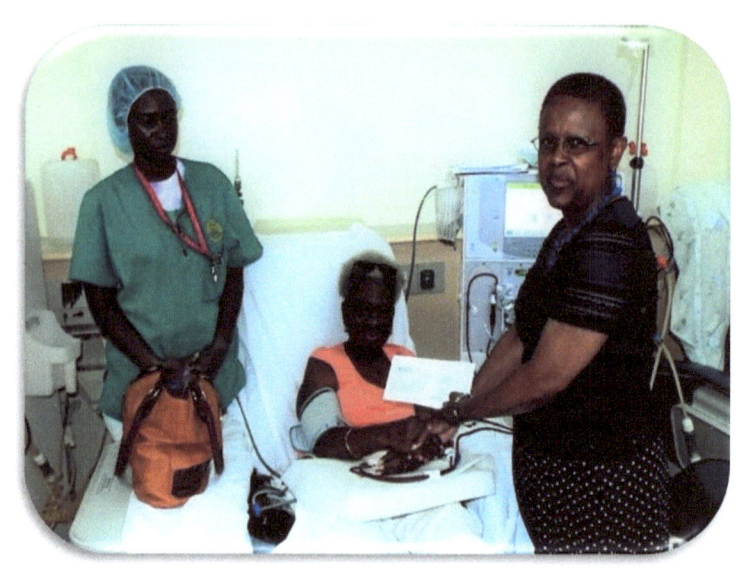

Beverley Knight receiving a donation for the dialysis unit from B.O.N.A QEH Barbados

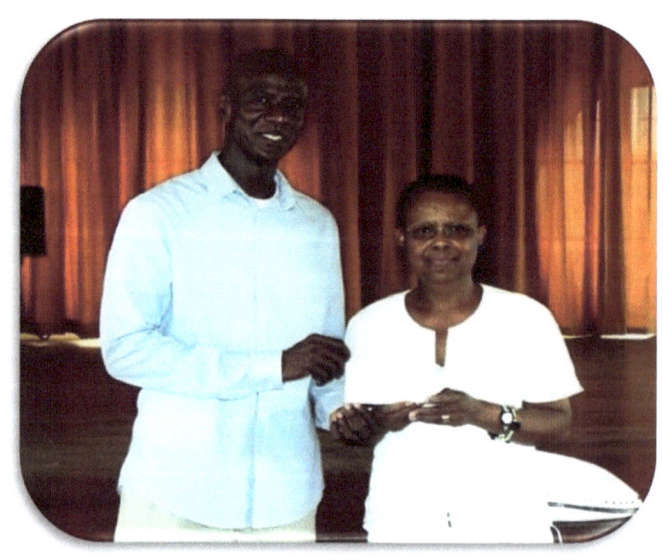

Mr. Jonathan Corbin, Principal of Princess Margaret Secondary School

Secondary School, receiving a cheque from B.O.N.A

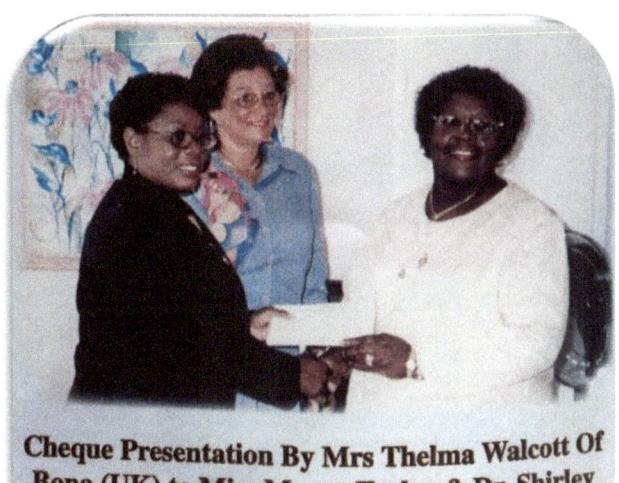

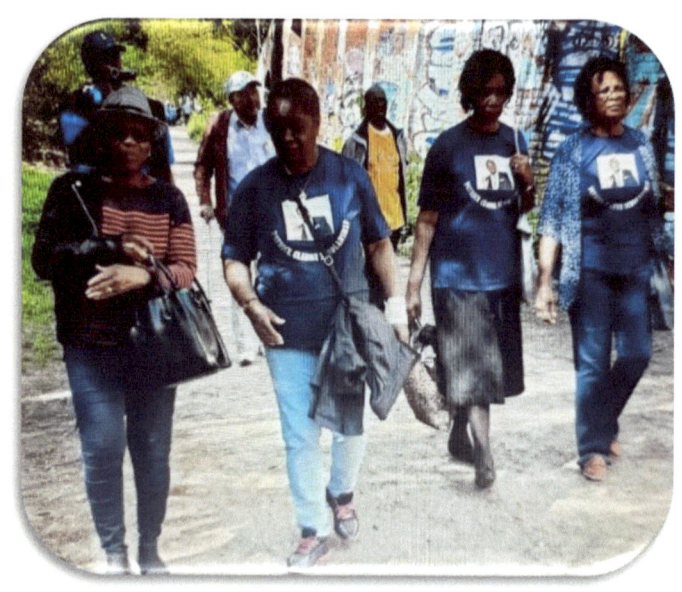

Walkers 2019 in foreground: Shermane, Carmita, Gloria, Waple
Background: Patrick, Harold, and Colvin

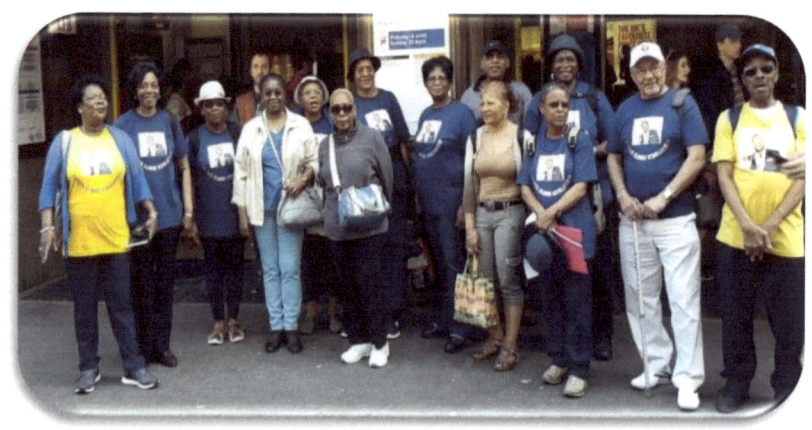

Gathering outside Holborn Station in preparation to visit parks around the City of London: Margaret, Gloria, Shermane,

Carmita, Gwendoline, Norma, Marie, Waple, Denise, Kenneth, Maria, Oriel, Harold and Colvin 2018

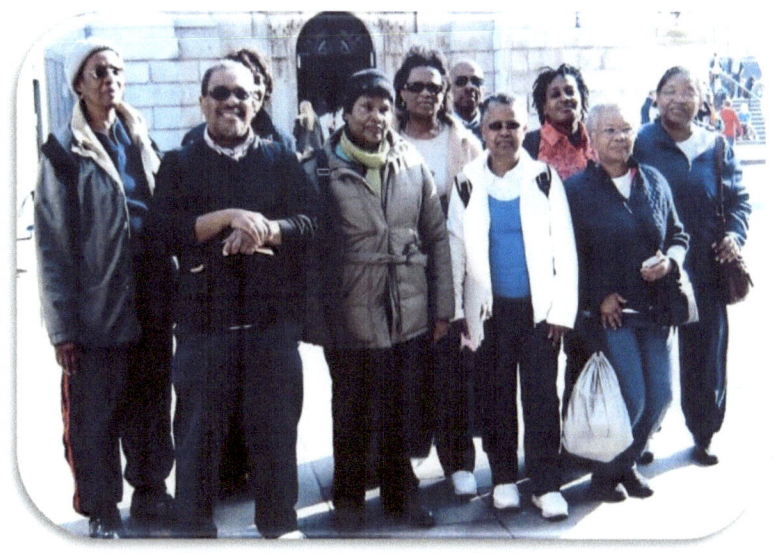

2015

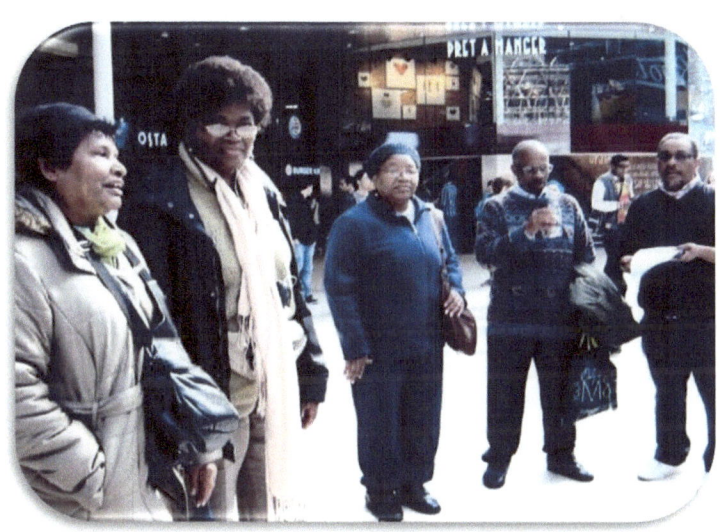

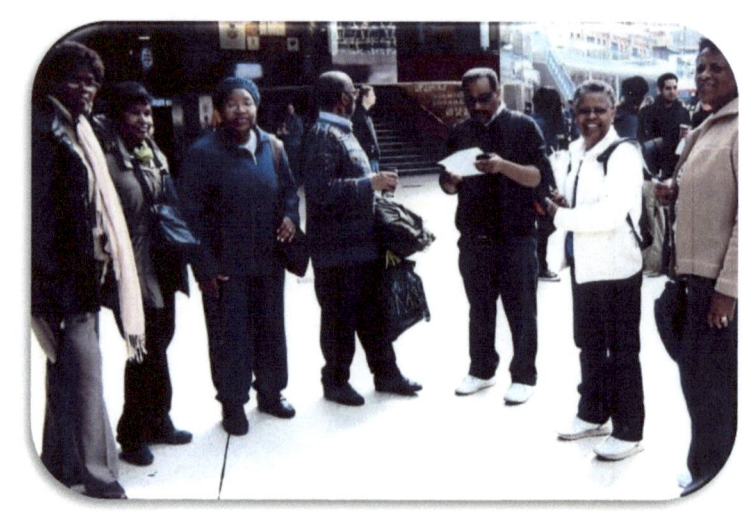

2014 x 2

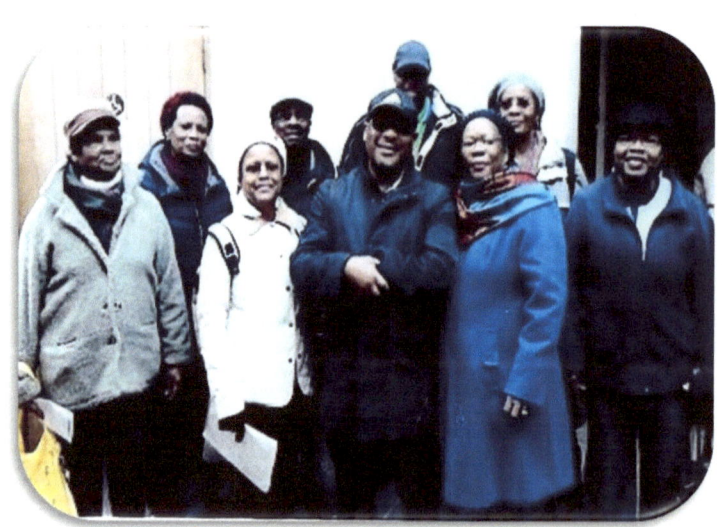

2015

Nita Joan Bynoe-Saul

I was selected to come to England through James Street Methodist Church, Bridgetown, Barbados, West Indies, where I used to worship every Sunday. The then Rev. Vivian recruited eligible girls to be trained as nurses.

I travelled on the fourteenth of November 1957 by ship, SS Hubert, one of three sister Portuguese ships, bringing recruits from Barbados to the UK. I arrived at Liverpool Docks, and then travelled to Waterloo Station, and on to Winchester Station in Hampshire where I started my training at St. Paul's Hospital. The Matron extended a very warm welcome to me and told me that I was very brave to travel all that way on my own.

On completion of my training, I was awarded the Sister Tutors Prize for my class work. From there, I went on to Harold Wood Hospital in Essex to be trained as a Student Nurse. Following this, I moved to St. Helier Hospital where I trained as a Midwife.

Overall, I enjoyed my training and career in the NHS, and made many friends at the various hospitals where I worked. I am now retired since 1995, and have no regrets and I also am at present a member of B.O.N.A.

My Journey Through the NHS and B.O.N.A by Phyllis Chase

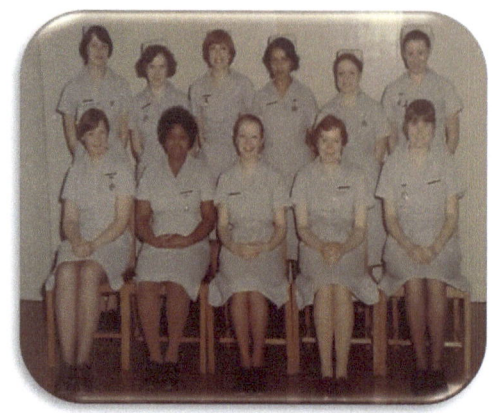

After hearing the news that England was desperate for nurses, I wrote a letter to Leavesden Hospital in Hertfordshire applying for a job. I was accepted with an offer to come to England and train as a RMNS nurse. I travelled to England in 1962 arriving at Leavesden Hospital on a Friday (fish and chip day). I was met and welcomed by the Home Sister. She said to me "leave your suitcase at the side by the door, we will go in and have supper". While I was eating in the dining room, I heard lots of loud voices giggling and chatting (apparently someone passed by and saw the name on the suitcase and 6 girls came to see if I was the new arrival). What a reunion I had. They were all my school mates, and I had no idea they were at this hospital. I was never lonely. I went on to do my training and enjoyed many years of living and working at Leavesden Hospital.

As time went by, I met other Barbadians and girls from other West Indian islands. I visited many places of interest and got to know England better.

I later worked at Edgware General, Mount Vernon and Harefield Hospital during the time of the first heart transplant, where my skills in reverse barrier nursing were put into practice. I also did further training at Watford General Hospital. I later left the NHS to join British Rail where I became an Accounts Clerk until I retired.

As years passed by, I joined various groups and became continually active in community projects and in 1996 the Barbados Government presented me with the High Commissioners Award for services to the community abroad.

I took up line dancing and tap dancing, tap being my favourite. For tap I passed all the exams I entered where I achieved high marks and I proudly display my medals on my mantelpiece to this day.

I came from a musical family back in Barbados and using that as a springboard I entertained regularly by singing, playing the piano and the guitar at various venues.

I joined B.O.N.A after being introduced by Pauline Sealey, a former President of B.O.N.A. I became a member of the choir. We sang at church services, weddings, funerals, and concerts. I supported them at outings, dinners, and some fundraising projects. I have performed at some of B.O.N.A's yearly concerts and, also at events at the Barbados High Commission.

I enjoy the friendship and love shown by the nurses in the group and I love sharing some of our favourite Bajan foods such as coconut bread, cod fish cakes and stew Conkies.

I cannot join B.O.N.A now as often as I would like to due to ill health, but they are always in my heart and in my thoughts. Love to all.

Tributes

Dalton McConney MBE, QPM

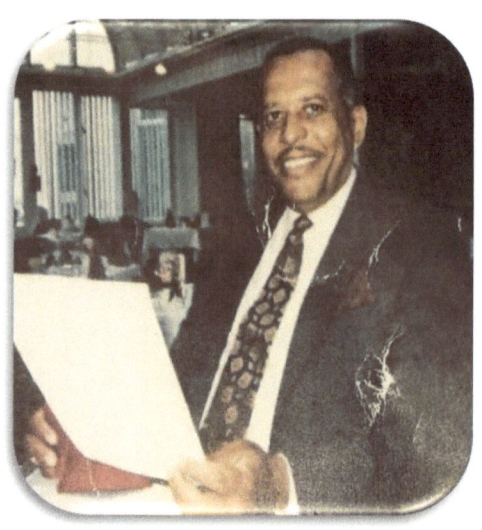

During the late nineteen fifties and early nineteen sixties the UK Government extended an invitation to the Caribbean young men and women to come to this country and fill some of the various occupations where work was available.

Many Barbadians (mostly men) answered this call but some of the "Jewels in our Crown" (our precious ladies) also answered that call, as the National Health Service desperately needed nurses for the depleted health service in the UK.

The stories of the reception and induction into their new careers are best told by those brave and resilient ladies who apparently endured some of the most hostile treatment. With true "Bajan Grit" they persevered and their contribution over the years was warmly acclaimed in the 70th Anniversary Celebration of the NHS in July 2018.

In 1994, some of the Stalwarts of the Barbadian UK nursing community, encouraged and supported by the then Deputy High Commissioner for Barbados Mr Owen Eversley, were instrumental in establishing the Barbados Overseas Nurses Association.

B.O.N.A's main goals were to use their expertise to establish a social and welfare mechanism for its members and to help and support through fundraising efforts, needy groups in this country and in Barbados.

There were difficulties along the way, but members then and now have worked with an unwavering and gratifying enthusiasm to achieve their goals.

Now a registered Charity, B.O.N.A. continues this work and 25 years of this service has not dimmed their dedication, compassion, and sacrifice.

This 25-year Anniversary Celebration is a tribute to those members who have given their service and earned the admiration and respect of the Barbados and UK communities. We salute those members who have gone to their eternal rest and in particular Patrick Clarke who tragically lost his life caring for the mentally ill.

I am deeply honoured to have been one of your patrons from the inception of the Association. Stella and I congratulate you all and wish you continued success in the future.

(Reprinted from the 25th. Anniversary Journal)

Herbert E Yearwood

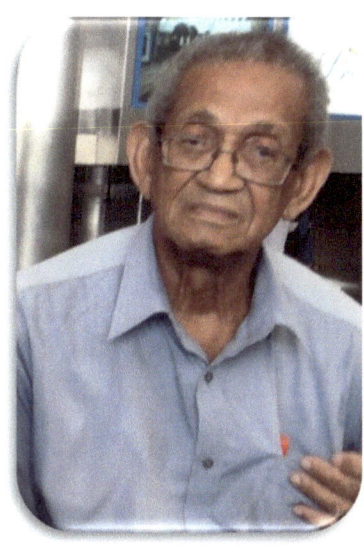

Deputy High Commissioner 1995-2008

During my tenure as Deputy High Commissioner for Barbados in the UK, The Barbados Nurses Association was one which stood out as a well organised and disciplined group It always appeared to be functioning in the interest of its members and promoting Barbados, their country of origin.

Its members always appeared eager to assist the High Commission in any way they could help.

The Nurses Association was immensely helpful when I coordinated the four Barbados and one Caribbean Expos between 1997 and 2006 and was always keen to support the Health and Welfare committee at the High Commission with their work.

The BONA choir was appreciated at Barbados Independence services or at any other Barbados functions where their melodious tones could be heard.

The Association was a shining example of what Barbadian Associations overseas should be.

Thanks for your service and contribution to the Barbados High

Commission and Barbadians in the UK during my tour of duty and may you continue to serve Barbados well.

Reverend David A. Hoyte

Whatever you do, work at it with all your heart, as working for the Lord, not for human masters, it is the Lord Christ you are serving. **Colossians 3:23-24**

I wish to extend my sincere best wishes to The Barbados Overseas Nurses Association (BONA) on the auspicious occasion of reaching twenty-five years as an organization. No doubt, there were challenges along the way, however with God as their guide, he has brought them thus far and will carry them on.

I especially admire the work that they do within the local community and Barbadian Diaspora. One such element was the formation of their choir, for which I had the privilege of leading for over 10 years. It was indeed a pleasure to lead them and I shall cherish the many memories of church services, concerts, and other occasions of which they performed at. They are a delightful group of dedicated persons, who over the years have remained true to their task, singing with great energy, zeal, and a tenacity for God. May B.O.N.A continue to go on, as long God's will endure for them. Every blessing.

Esther Holmes, MBE (Friend and Supporter of BONA since 1994)

Barbados Nurses in the UK are a true reflection of our motto "Pride and Industry".

First, let me thank you for raising the profile of Barbados, internationally. Your selfless contribution to the sick and vulnerable within a fledgling NHS of the 1950s/60s is legendary. You left Barbados as young women (mainly) at a time when Barbados was still a British colony or just emerging as a nation. You were nurtured, developed, and educated under the British flag. Your philosophy on life and your Christian Faith coupled with your unique qualities of perseverance, empathy and good old common sense have brought you through high times of great personal successes and achievements and low periods of incredible difficulties. But now we must look forward to the next 25 years and beyond. Several contributions to this 25th Anniversary booklet have given interesting insights into possible future direction.

They have said:

"<u>Our Partners</u> were the backbone of our efforts without their support our good work would not have been possible."

"<u>My late husband</u> shared our domestic roles; he took care of our sons".

"I had a daughter but continued my career with good support <u>from my husband</u>"

"Personally, I thought (initially) that husbands and partners were there to support BONA with the lifting and carrying, but now I am BONA's dancing instructor, art teacher, secretary and member of BONA's Choir (the Bass duo)."

"I met my wife at one of BONA's dances. I now help to organise a number of B.O.N.A events as a member of their social committee."

Several BONA's members have highlighted the support and encouragement that they have received from their husband/partners, particularly with the difficulties of raising a young family and serving within the NHS, at the same time.

The full impact of the extended family contribution, in this context, has not yet been fully assessed.

BONA's 25th anniversary celebration is a timely reminder of the number of "unsung heros"[9] who have contributed for many years, to BONA's success.

Anthony Sandiford, Chair WIFFA

It is with great pleasure that I, on the behalf of members of WIFFA have been asked to write this tribute to Barbados Overseas Nurses Association B.O.N.A.

Over the years B0NA has proven that coming together as a group creates strength among that group and certain benefits to the Community. As the title suggests many of the Association's members and affiliates would have had a long and distinguished career in the field of nursing, hence their combined expertise would be second to none.

Dedication in the field of nursing even long after retirement is a true testament to their care and consideration of vulnerable persons in the society. BONA is not only about nursing and nursing skills but has focused on the improvement of knowledge and wellbeing of its members and the wider community.

The Association has also showcased other skills such as singing, dancing, poetry reading and the arrangement of other educational and social activities to build up a portfolio which it shares with the wider community.

The longevity and success of the Association can be attributed to the leadership, dedication, and commitment of the management over the years, who must be congratulated for successfully negotiating many of the pitfalls that often beset most Associations and sometimes bring about its downfall. Pitfalls such as dealing with disgruntled members, resistance to new changes, lack of focus, sickness, death, and repatriations are just a few.

May you continue to build on the solid foundation which has been laid and ensure that Barbados Overseas Nurses Association will be remembered long after the founding members have passed.

Congratulations

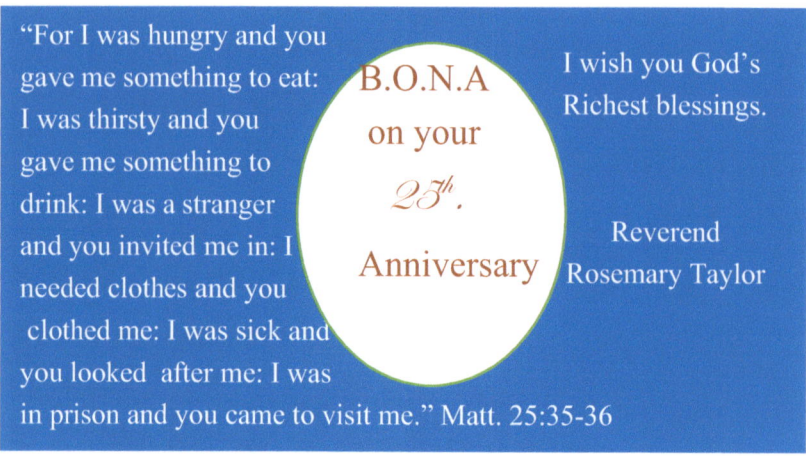

Keep up the good work (2019)

Below are selections of the arts and crafts unit in B.O.N.A.

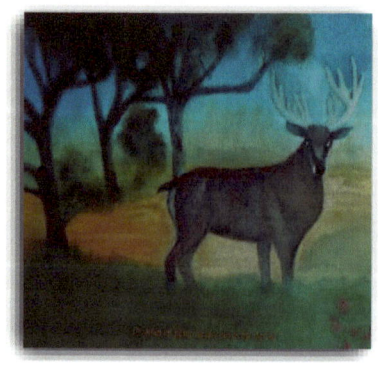

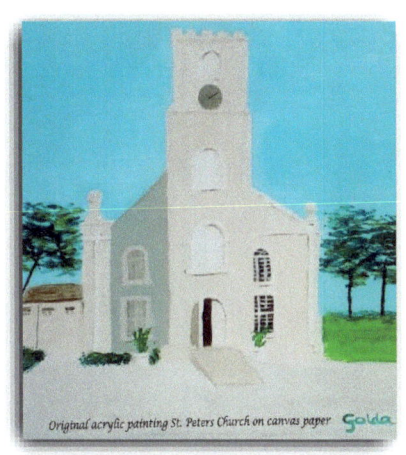

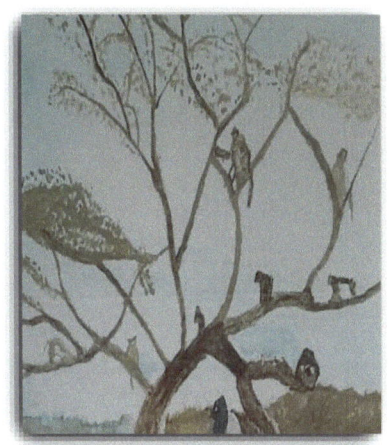

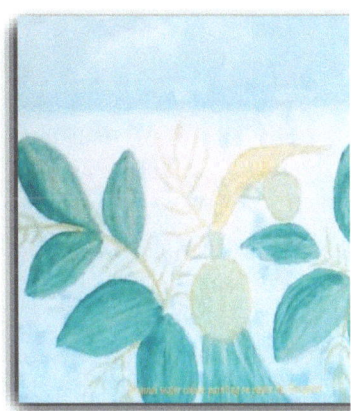

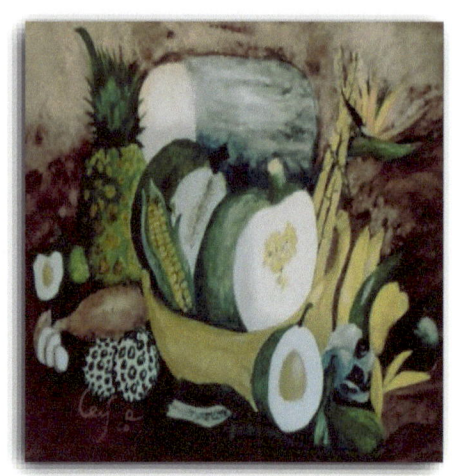

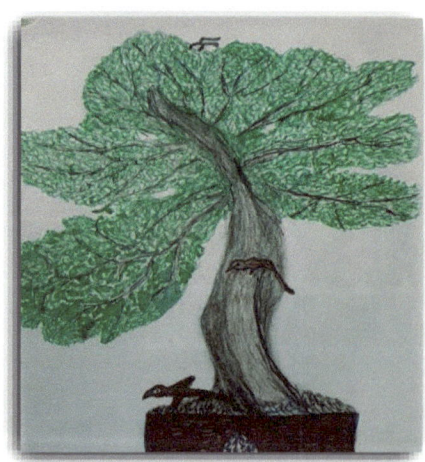

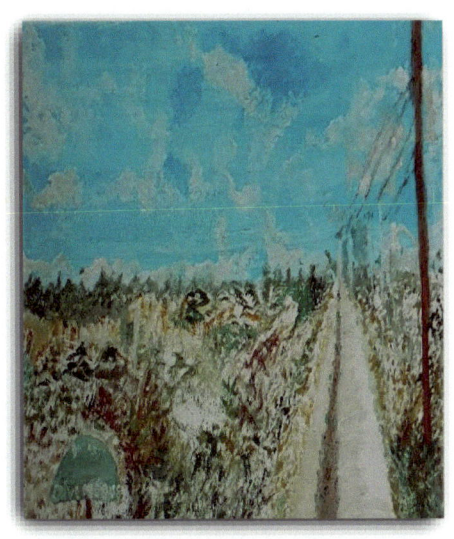
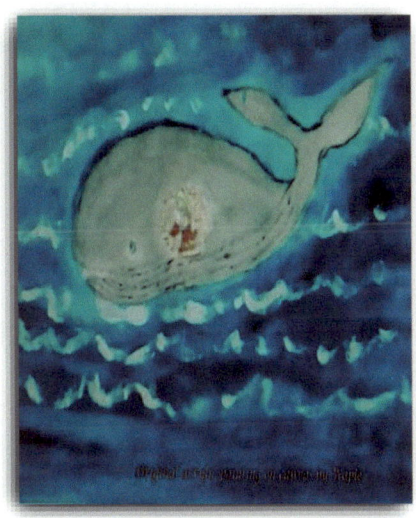

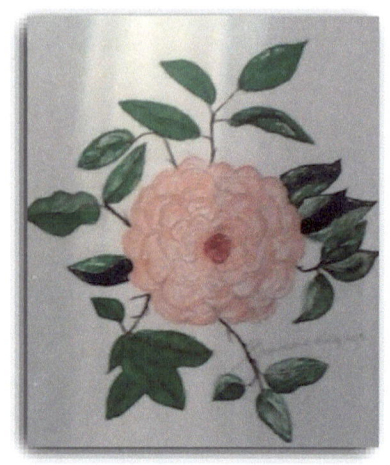 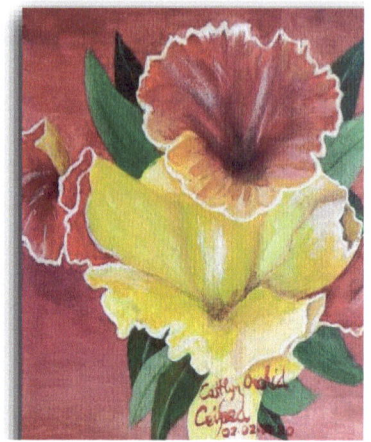

The Arts Class has been fantastic from day one and the samples of their tremendous talents displayed on this page exemplify their steadfast commitment and endurance. The association is forever grateful for their efforts and thank them, namely Ceifred (Instructor), Harold, Colvin, Waple, Margaret, Jean, Golda, Carmita and Shermane.

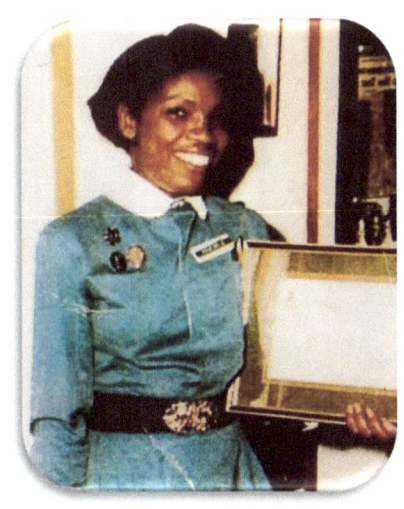

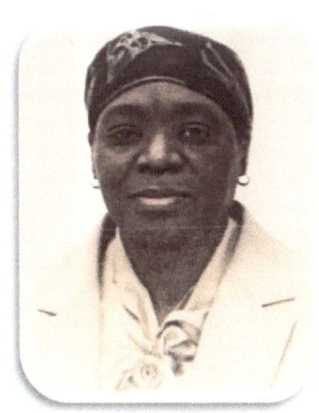 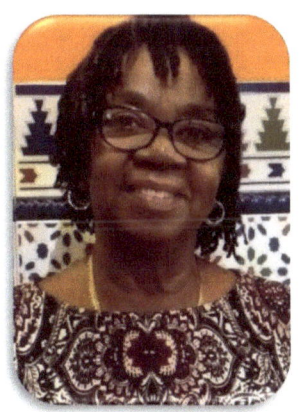

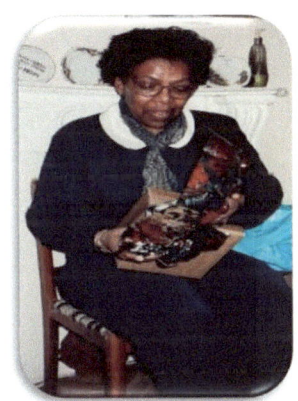 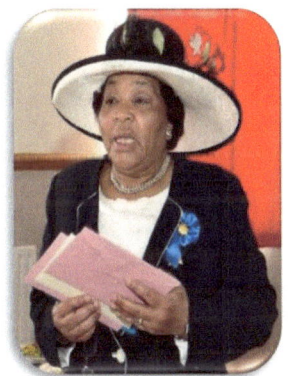

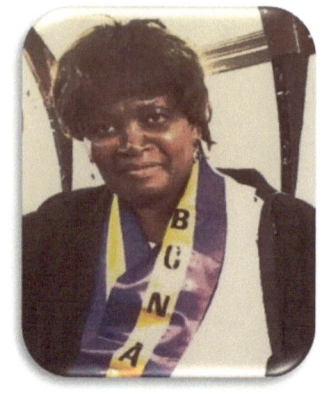 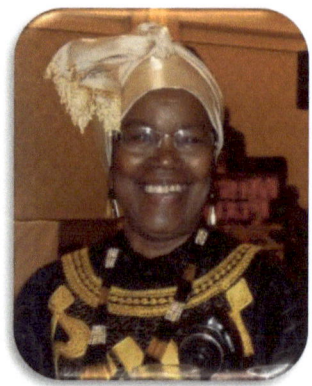

Top: Shermane Peters, President
Former Presidents: Pauline Sealy*
Barbara Brewster
Eudese Haynes* and Cynthia Coker
Oriel Weekes, Yvonne Goodman*.

deceased

Acknowledgement: Oriel Weekes (Founder Member & PP), Shermane Peters (P), Barbara Brewster (PP) MBE JP, Norma & Gladstone Redwood-Sawyerr, Marie Greenridge, Angela Alleyne, Margaret Morris-Springer (VP), Maria Y. Layne-Springer, Gloria Gittins, Ceifred Goodman Julia Alleyne, Dalton McConney MBE QPM, Harold Springer, Isalene Carter, Carmita Neblett, Rev Rosemary Taylor Chaplain, Golda Griffiths, Esther Holmes MBE, Rev Jackie Cockfield, Jean Millar, Herbert "Herbie" Yearwood,
Anthony Sandiford, Rev. David Hoyte

Present Members

Norma Alfee	Carmen Doughlin
Julia Alleyne	Correl Goodridge-Felce
Angel Alleyne	Isalene Carter
Grace Alleyne	Phyllis Chase
Faustina Alleyne	Ceifred Goodman
Waple Baird	Golda Griffith
Millicent Batson	Monica Gordon
Barbara Brewster	Gloria Gittins
Victor Brewster	Marie Greenidge
Cynthia Coker	Newla Greenidge
Shirley Clarke	Grace Hamblin
Rev Jackie Cockfield	Ermine Hunte

Irma Inniss
Clovine Morris
Hamilton Marshall
Hammington Marshall, (H)
Yvonne Norris
Carmita Neblett
Margaret Morris-Springer
Colvin Springer
Anne Okokon
Shermane Peters
Gladstone Redwood-Sawyerr
Norma Redwood-Sawyerr
Clarene Russell
Shirlene Rudder (H)
Joan Saul
Joan Tull
Eurla White
Oriel Weekes
Patrick Weekes
Conchita Webbe
Lorraine Whitehall
Ralph Waithe
Gloria Wilson
Norma Johnson
Maria Layne-Springer
Kenneth Phillips
Elaine Joseph
Marcia Jones-Warner

Anderson Seale, (H)
Harold Springer
Cecelia Rodrigues

EXECUTIVE OFFICERS & COMMITTEE
2004 – 2020

PATRONS: BARBADOS HIGH COMMISSIONER
& MR. DALTON Mc CONNEY MBE QPM

CHAPLAIN: Rev. ROSEMARY TAYLOR

PRESIDENTS
Mrs. BARBARA BREWSTER
Mrs. CYNTHIA COKER
MS ORIEL WEEKES
Mrs. YVONNE GOODMAN
Mrs. SHERMANE PETERS

VICE PRESIDENTS

Dr NOLA ISMAIEL
Mrs. PATRICIA SPRINGER
Mrs. JEAN GAY*
MARGARET MORRIS-SPRINGER

SECRETARIES
Mrs. MARIE GREENIDGE
Mr. CEIFRED GOODMAN

ASSISTANT SECRETARIES

Mrs. ANNA OKOKON

TREASURERS

MS JULIA ALLEYNE

Mrs. MARIA LAYNE-SPRINGER

ASSISTANT TREASURER

Mrs. MARGARET MORRIS-SPRINGER

SOCIAL CO-ODINATORS

Norma Redwood-Sawyerr

Margaret Morris-Springer

Yvonne Goodman*

Harold Springer

COMMITTEE MEMBERS

Shermane Peters

Margaret Morris-Springer

Ceifred Goodman

Maria Layne-Springer

Harold Springer

Hamilton Marshall

Oriel Weekes

Gwendoline Joseph

Waple Baird

Monica Gordon

Hamilton Marshall

Gloria Gittens
Marie Greenidge
Colvin Springer
Conchita Webbe
Newla Greenidge
Yvonne Norris
Golda Griffith
Norma Alfee

CARE & SUPPORT CO-ORDINATORS
Millicent Batson
Gwendoline Joseph

Choir CO-ORDINATORS
Ceifred Goodman

Oriel Weekes

Appendix

Barbados Overseas Nurses Association was founded in 1994 with the aim of uniting nurses from Barbados to aid each other in issues of interest while finding their way in the United Kingdom.

MEMBERSHIP IS BY INTRODUCTION AND IS ALSO OPENED TO ALL PEOPLE OF CARIBBEAN ORIGIN.

B.O.N.A governing body consists of a President, V-President, Treasurer and Secretary, together with the Co-Ordinator of the Education, Care and Support, Social and Choir Committees plus four co-opted members, elected and appointed by the membership at the Annual General Meeting in June.

Mission Statement:

To plan carefully, respond appropriately, monitor consistently, and evaluate to realise our vision, and achieve the aims and objectives.

Our Vision:

Promoting a better world by being a part of the solution.

Barbados Overseas Nurses Association became a Reg. Charity No. 1142895 and a Limited Company by Guarantee No. 7564758 in 2011 to extend the work of giving in all areas of need. Organizations who benefit from our efforts are the Barbados Diabetic Association, Barbados Council for Disability, Alzheimer's Society UK and Barbados, African Caribbean Leukemia Trust (ACLT) Barbados Kidney Association and the Princess Margaret Secondary School. We also gave one-off donations to deserving causes such as the Haitian earthquake disaster, and the Grenadian hurricane relief.

Recreation:

Exercise classes, Line Dancing, painting and other arts and crafts activities every Wednesday morning at 11am are proving phenomenally successful. We also regularly arrange other cultural events in the
community.

Our choir boasts a healthy 27 members including the organist and choir master, regularly answers the many requests to sing at various functions.

There are film nights at regular intervals during the year, storytelling, art exhibitions and lunch breaks.

We also have an annual sponsored walk as a special fundraiser for nominated charity.

Our annual Thanksgiving Service is held on the second Sunday in May and is always well attended. Our Christmas celebration is highlighted by "Nine Lessons and Carols" performed by the choir and the other members.

Aims:

Support members socially, emotionally, and educationally. Engage proactively with young people through appropriate forums such as seminars and conferences. Identify medical, educational, social, and recreational projects in Barbados, Eastern Caribbean, and the UK.

Build effective working relationships within the community and other Associations.

Raising awareness in the membership of health issues, especially in the elderly.

The remarkable stories in this book represent a historical account of the unsung, and perhaps likely forgotten, heroes and heroines of the many young men and women, mainly Barbadians, who gladly responded to the anxious call of the "Mother Country" (UK) to serve in the depleted NHS which was desperately in need of a workforce for the many hospitals across the country…as nurses, they worked with an unwavering and gratifying enthusiasm to meet the demands despite facing hostile treatment in some cases…In the words of the first President, the late Pauline Sealy, one of six pioneers who started the Barbados Overseas Nurses Association, affectionately called "B.O.N.A": "I'd like the memory of me to be a happy one, and to leave an afterglow of smiles when my life is done." A fitting tribute for the organisation and the members, who have dedicated themselves in fundraising to help the community and other deserving causes in the UK, African Caribbean Leukaemia Trust (LCLT) and Barbados, Grenada and other Caribbean countries struck by hurricanes, earthquakes and other disasters. The fundraising efforts comprised of various recreational activities, Line Dancing in tune with healthy lifestyle, Sponsored Walks, Art, producing a yearly calendar and exhibitions. There is also a successful choir of 25 persons, performing at various events across the nation, raising funds. Dedication in the field of nursing even long after retirement is a true testament to their care and consideration of vulnerable persons in society. BONA is not only about nursing and nursing skills but has focused on the improvement of knowledge and wellbeing of its members and the wider community, and has also showcased other skills such as singing, dancing, poetry reading and the arrangement of other educational and social activities to build up a portfolio which it shares with the wider community, especially the youth.

www.ingramcontent.com/pod-product-compliance
Lightning Source LLC
Chambersburg PA
CBHW040219220526
45473CB00001B/52